Torsten Schwalm Modern Tilt Table Testing and Non-Invasive Monitoring

"Those who suffer from frequent
and severe fainting often die suddenly."

Hippocrates, Aphorisms 2.41, 1000 B.C.E.

Torsten Schwalm

Modern Tilt Table Testing and Non-Invasive Monitoring

Traditional and Innovative Applications in Theory and Practice

Foreword by R. A. Kenny

ABW · Wissenschaftsverlag

ABW Wissenschaftsverlag GmbH
Kurfürstendamm 57
10707 Berlin
Germany
www.abw-verlag.de

Sandgasse 3
3652 Leiben
Austria

Dr. med. Dipl. med. inf. (FH) Torsten Schwalm
Greifswalder Str. 208b
10405 Berlin
Germany
t.schwalm@gmx.de

Klinikum Frankfurt/Oder
Müllroser Chaussee 7
15236 Frankfurt/Oder
Germany
t.schwalm.km@klinikumffo.de

English translation: Manuela Schatz
Cover design: Karla Detlefsen, Rudolf Hübler; Berlin
Cover figure: The figure on the cover shows a 3-dimensional diagram of physiological behavior of sympathetic and vagal frequency components of cardiovascular autonomous heart rate control during different stages of a tilt table testing procedure (see Fig. 7, p. 66)
Set by: Type-Design, Berlin
Printed and bound by: DZA Druckerei zu Altenburg GmbH, Altenburg

ISBN-10: 3-936072-47-7
ISBN-13: 978-3-936072-47-1
Printed in Germany

Contents

Foreword

Maimonides, as far back as the 12th century, recognized the impact of unexplained syncope on the individual and society – *"only if one knows the cause of syncope will he be able to recognize its onset and combat the cause"*.

Physicians have long since struggled with this paroxysmal symptom which encroaches on the clinical practice of many specialties including family practice, the emergency room, neurology, geriatric medicine and psychiatry. Syncope is prevalent in all age groups from paediatrics through to old age.

Sir Thomas Lewis in his classical essay on vaso-vagal syncope in 1932 systematically characterized, for the first time, its clinical and haemodynamic features. Yet a diagnostic test for this common symptom was not available for a further 60 years until the advent of tilt table testing.

Tilt table testing is attractive because it is a simple, non-invasive test available to the wider medical community, which has further evolved with the development of simultaneous non-invasive methods for monitoring the cardiovascular and autonomic nervous system. Clarity for diagnostic indications, interpretation of haemodynamic and neural data and interpretation of test outcomes has to date been lacking. This new text makes significant in-roads into this uncertainty. It amalgamates extant information on all relevant clinical and research aspects of the test leaving no stone unturned and provides an easy to read, easy to access, timely and comprehensive overview. Clinicians who deal with syncope, irrespective of their sub-specialty, will readily apply this information to their daily practice.

Professor Rose Anne Kenny
Professor of Clinical Gerontology, Trinity College Dublin
Visiting Professor of Cardiovascular Research,
University of Newcastle-upon-Tyne

Preface

It was whilst researching the pathogenesis of hypertension that I recognized the need for a technique that allowed simultaneous non-invasive, continuous monitoring of both peripheral vascular resistance and activity of the autonomic nervous system. From this evolved the concept of the complex non-invasive monitoring of hemodynamic and autonomic functions. Supported by the Austrian Science Funds (FWF Austria), notably the funding program "Sonderforschungsbereich 007", we developed a prototype of the Task Force Monitor, which comprised a combination of then commercially available devices that monitored hemodynamic parameters and a program for beat-to-beat evaluation of hemodynamic and autonomic parameters. Only a few experiments (e.g., hemodynamic and autonomic effects of insulin-induced hypoglycemia or of vasodilator infusion) were necessary to confirm that this type of monitoring would eventually be indispensable to clinical medicine as well as to physiology and pharmacology.

During the subsequent years, this prototype, notably in combination with tilt testing, was successfully used for the diagnosis of hemodynamic and autonomic disorders. Eventually it was replaced by the "Task Force Monitor". This device was developed in a small research laboratory in our hospital as part of several diploma theses. Since then it has become a worldwide success, and an indispensable tool for physicians who deal with hemodynamics and the autonomic nervous system. This device has led to a new era for medical practice and research. In the early stages of the Task Force Monitor it was necessary to analyze many print-report-pages full of complex information in order to obtain a definite diagnosis, but since then we have enabled the user to evaluate and analyze all obtained parameters within mere seconds by means of the "one-page-report". However, the interpretation of this novel technology requires experience and knowledge of the methodology that is not currently being taught in medical schools. This compendium offers a comprehensive review of the functions of the autonomic nervous system, and its case studies illustrate the significance of monitoring hemodynamic and autonomic parameters. The present compendium is to be recommended to all those who have to deal with syncope, hemodynamics and the autonomic nervous system. It is anticipated that this book will broaden the use of this method and move it firmly into routine clinical practice.

University Professor Dr. Falko Skrabal
Head of the Department of Internal Medicine
and Medical Director of the Hospital Barmherzige Brüder
(Teaching Hospital of the Medical University of Graz)

Author's preface

To address the wide variety of diagnostic, therapeutic and economic issues that surround the symptom complex of syncope, the concept of a "syncope facility" has emerged [34,154].

The current suboptimal management of syncope will be improved by the use of well-structured, algorithm-orientated diagnostic pathways in specialized syncope facilities with ambulatory patient care, appropriate core equipment and the ready availability of additional diagnostic methods.

The undirected use of diagnostic tests in syncope management is not only disadvantageous to patients but also financially uneconomical. Studies estimate [49,242] that the diagnostic costs related to syncope range between $5,000 and $16,000 per patient. Despite this extensive use of diagnostic tools, no definitive diagnosis is established in up to 50% of cases [49,82].

Tilt table testing, impedance cardiography and continuous non-invasive blood pressure monitoring are devices that play a key role in cardiology and related specialities. Developments in this area, particularly with regard to measuring technologies and software, provide insights into the complex processes of hemodynamic functions and cardiovascular autonomic control. Often, "syncope" is the presentation of an underlying abnormality, and as such the investigation of syncope involves almost all medical specialities, and hence requires a multidisciplinary approach.

The theory and practice of modern tilt table testing and non-invasive monitoring for diagnostic purposes are the central themes of the following compendium. The potential applications now far exceed the original areas of use and tilt table testing now plays a part in the development of new and innovative therapeutic approaches.

While part I provides a review of the theoretical principles of syncope, tilt table testing and allied diagnostic fields, part II focuses on providing practical explanations of the multifaceted applications, with real-life examples being presented in part III.

Torsten Schwalm Berlin, January, 2006

Acknowledgements

I want to thank Ms. Doris Flotzinger and Ms. Sara Alkan for their unwearying support and for their excellent cooperation, as well as Dr. Axel Bedürftig for his "publishing enthusiasm". I am also thankful for Ms. Julia Newton's editorial support, which has been very valuable for the success of this project. And last but not least I want to mention my wife Gudrun, whose untiring patience I will always appreciate.

Introductory remarks

We want to apologize for the fact that some of the diagrams and charts in Chapters 2 and 3 contain display texts in German. In fact, these diagrams were generated during patient work-ups in a German hospital, and thus the software-language was set to "German".

1 Theoretical review

1.1 The introduction of tilt table testing

60 years ago the first study examining the physiological and pathophysiological effects of orthostatic stress by tilt table testing [8] was published.

In 1986, Kenny et al. [151] observed an abnormal response to orthostatic provocation using tilt table testing in 10 out of 15 patients diagnosed with syncope of uncertain cause and established this technique for the diagnosis of vasovagal syncope.

Subsequently the procedure was refined to come close to becoming a "gold standard" for the diagnosis of vasovagal syncope. Assessment strategies have been modified repeatedly, which is reflected in the wide variety of available protocols. Tilt test duration, angle of tilting, importance of and possible use of provocative stimuli are issues that are still scientifically discussed.

But even more important than these modifications and developments is the key role that the tilt table procedure plays in the differential diagnosis of unexplained faints and syncope, as exemplified in several expert consensus documents [16] and guidelines [33,34].

The combination of tilt table testing with non-invasive techniques such as continuous (beat-to-beat) blood pressure measurement, recording of hemodynamic parameters and data of the autonomic nervous system, has simplified traditional diagnostic approaches and has also considerably extended diagnostic application.

1.2 The use of tilt table testing in the management of syncope

1.2.1 Definition

Syncope is defined as a transient, self-limiting loss of consciousness caused by global cerebral hypoperfusion, accompanied by a loss of voluntary muscle tone as well as spontaneous recovery when lying supine. Syncope is not a disease but a symptom complex.

In this review, an episode of syncope is described when matching the above, simple definition. In many publications, the clinical features do not correspond to the restricted specific definition. For instance, a loss of consciousness due to hypoglycemia is not a syncopal episode, because recovery does not occur after a change in posture, but rather by administration of glucose.

1.2.2 Symptomatology

Syncope onset is usually without warning, its progress rapid and the subsequent recovery prompt and without residual deficits. A syncopal episode generally is of less than 20 seconds in duration. In the study of Lempert [127] the symptom duration averaged 12 seconds.

Syncope is associated with a wide variety of clinical manifestations. Clonic movements may result in a misdiagnosis of epilepsy but are in fact caused by global cerebral hypoperfusion and not due to excessive cerebroelectric activity and neural discharge. The term "convulsive" syncope describes this condition. In some cases the presyncopal phase is associated with symptoms like light-headedness, sweating, nausea, weakness and hyperventilation, a sensation of physical alienation or visual disturbances preceding actual syncope [105,158,324].

1.2.3 Classification

There are a number of different classifications for the clinical picture of syncope which are dependent upon the underlying disease, pathophysiology [33], or the hemodynamic patterns during, or prior to, syncope during passive orthostasis. Abnormal responses during tilt table testing can be classified broadly into four categories (Fig. 1). The first category describes a classical vasovagal reaction associated with the sudden occurrence of hypotension with, or without, bradycardia. Patients affected are typically young and otherwise healthy. The second category is called the "dysautonomic" response type, which is characterized by a continuous, concurrent decrease in systolic and diastolic blood pressure, often in correlation with autonomic dysfunctions such as abnormal perspiration, impaired micturition or defecation. Patients affected are in general older, and considerably more afflicted. The third category is associated with increasing tachycardia and more or less stable blood pressure and is called Postural Orthostatic Tachycardia Syndrome (see Chapter 1.2.3.5.3). Finally the fourth category is characterized by a physiological response pattern, where in spite of simultaneous clinical symptoms of syncope or presyncope there is no hemodynamic change. This pattern is consistent with an underlying psychiatric illness such as a panic disorder or depression.

Sutton [306] proposed a classical classification based upon heart rate and blood pressure behavior during tilt-induced syncope

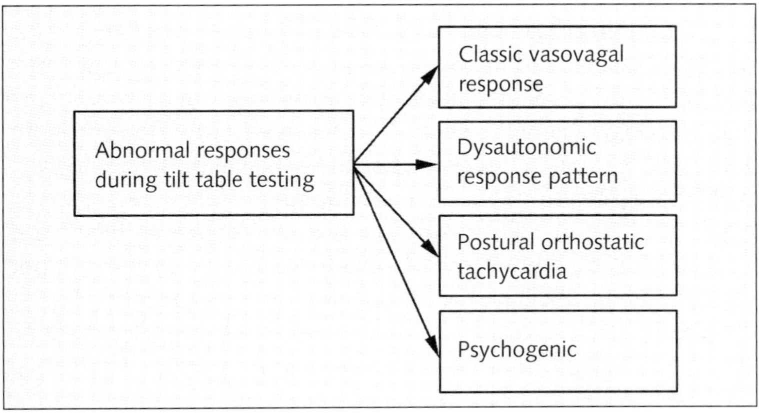

Figure 1 Classification of abnormal responses during tilt table testing.

known as the VASIS classification. Brignole [36] postulated a classification based upon hemodynamic changes during the presyncopal phase (Tables 7 and 8, Chapter 2.2.2.1.1).

Potential etiological factors for syncope can also be classified into four categories (Fig. 2). However, it is important to distinguish between actual syncope and symptoms mimicking syncope, where clinical features do not correspond to the definition described above and which are generally associated with a different etiology.

Syncopes can be assigned to two main groups. The majority are the neurally mediated reflex syncopes, followed by those with syncope of unknown etiology [146]. The use of new diagnostic devices, particularly tilt table testing, can considerably reduce the latter group with 50–66% of those who would previously have been diagnosed as syncope of unclear origin diagnosed as neurally mediated reflex syncope. The latter diagnostic group is followed in order of frequency by syncopes of cardiac, neurological and psychogenic origin.

1.2.3.1 Category 1: Neurally mediated reflex syncope

1.2.3.1.1 Pathophysiology

On assuming the upright posture there is a gravitational shift of 300–800 ml of blood to the lower limbs followed by a decrease in stroke volume and arterial blood pressure.

Interruption of cerebral blood flow of 6–8 seconds [275], a decrease in arterial systolic blood pressure of 60 mmHg [290] or a 20 percent drop in cerebral oxygen delivery, are usually sufficient to lead to loss of consciousness. Via pressor receptors located in the aortic arc, the regulatory centers of the brain stem that are responsible for the efferent regulation of sympathetic functions are stimulated, resulting in vasoconstriction and an increase in heart rate. The purpose of this reflex is to maintain arterial systemic blood pressure at a sufficient threshold. Information about the state of the cardiac contractility is via non-myelinated, so-called C-fibers which send signals to the vagus nucleus which is located in the nucleus tractus solitarii of the brain stem. In the case of left ventricular hypercontractility [149,245,289] induced by prolonged standing, it comes to an efferent counterregulatory response via the cardiac fibers of the vagal nerve. This counterregulatory response is associated with a decrease in heart rate and cardiac inotropism as well as a withdrawal of sympathetic tone. This mechanism is a physiologically finely tuned reflex arc which is pathologically altered in patients susceptible to neurally mediated reflex syncope. Symptoms of this pathologically altered regulatory reflex are excessive bradycardia/asystole and/or hypotension. Bradycardia is a vagal mechanism and can be remedied by administration of atropine [180], hypotension is caused by withdrawal of sympathetic tone [218] and is resistant to treatment by anticholinergics or electric stimulation [299].

Another mechanism that can cause syncope is the sudden post-exercise withdrawal of sympathetic tone, whilst peripheral vasodilatation, due to increased limb perfusion, still persists.

Irrespective of the etiology of syncope, hypoperfusion of the cerebral cortex, or of the reticular activating system, is generally considered to be the common final phase.

Hypercontractility induced by the sympathetic nervous system has been a hypothesis that is controversial and not generally accepted [129]. An important counterargument is that patients whose autonomic cardiac innervation has been removed completely or to a great extent by dissection of the ascending aorta when undergoing coronary bypass surgery, cardiac valve replacement or heart transplantation [283], can still be afflicted by neurally mediated reflex syncope. Since mechanoreceptors have also been detected in the pulmonic arteries, the hypothesis of hypercontractility induced by the sympathetic nervous system cannot be disproved completely beyond dispute. In experimental studies imitating the reflex arc, with withdrawal of cardiac preload, only a slight stimulation of afferent nerves was observed [328].

Numerous authors have assumed that the cause of altered cardiovascular autonomic function lies in the brain itself. A further hypothesis assumes its origin is in an imbalance of the levels of cerebral neurotransmitters serotonin [115], vasopressin [129] and endorphin [190]. Clinical features of anxiety-induced (emotionally mediated) syncope support this theory. Emotional stimuli can trigger excessive bradycardia and hypotension via central neurotransmitters like beta-endorphin or serotonin [191]. Syncope triggered by pain, e.g. in the setting of trigeminal or glossopharyngeal neuralgia [33], also belong to this category.

The occurrence of cerebral vasospasms might also play a significant role in the multifactorial pathophysiology of syncope. Recent findings using transcranial Doppler ultrasonography [7,291] in patients with a positive response to tilt table testing support this hypothesis.

Patients with an abnormal electroencephalographic response in the left hemisphere subsequently had a positive response to tilt table testing, whereas this pattern was not observed in patients with negative response [52]. Without wanting to suggest a specific underlying mechanism, these findings would point towards changed neuronal activity.

An area of particular interest is baroreceptor reflex behavior in patients with syncope. The sensitivity of the reflex arc (baroreflex sensitivity/BRS) varies depending upon the specific syncopal pattern. Flevari [93] describes reduced baroreflex sensitivity in patients with syncope, as well as disaggregation of the baroreceptor-induced heart rate increase, which in healthy individuals is finally balanced, as well as reduction of peripheral blood flow due to vasoconstriction. In patients showing vasodepressor patterns a global impaired baroreflex sensitivity is the dominating feature, whereas in patients with cardioinhibitory responses there exists an instability in the balance between heart rate variability and peripheral vasoconstriction. It is possible that not all baroreceptor reflex functions are affected equally. Studies suggest disturbances in the regulation of baroreceptor reflex sequences responsible for its deactivation ("down-events", i.e. drop in blood pressure and reduction of RR-intervals [see Chapter 1.5.1]) in patients susceptible to vasovagal syncopes [261].

Samniah [279] observed a constant reduction of baroreflex sensitivity without adequate compensatory responses to prolonged orthostatic stress in patients with tilt-induced syncopal spells. A sudden and inadequate adjustment of rated values in the sense of a "resetting" [226] triggers the withdrawal of sympathetic tone regardless of hypotension.

However, today, the exact mechanism still remains unclear, even 70 years after introduction of the term "vasovagal syncope" [180].

1.2.3.1.2 Classification of neurally mediated reflex syncope

Neurally mediated reflex syncope can be classified into three subcategories:

1. Vasovagal syncope
2. Carotid sinus syncope
3. Situational syncope

Generally, in addition to the causes of syncope described above, vasovagal syncope is the most frequently encountered cause of a syncopal episode, whereas carotid sinus syncope occurs only rarely.

Dependent upon the pathophysiology [33], or the hemodynamics during, or prior to, syncope [36, 306] vasovagal syncope can be subdivided further (Tables 7 and 8; Chapter 2.2.2.1.1).

The spontaneous symptomatic syndrome of carotid sinus hypersensitivity is found in 1% of all syncopal episodes [311], but symptomatic hemodynamic responses to carotid sinus massage are significantly more frequent. Various studies report that they account for 26–60% of unexplained syncopes [37,104,133,211,320].

The carotid sinus reflex is a reflex arc that arises from pressor receptors located in the carotid bifurcation with afferent fibers terminating in the cardiovascular centers located in the rhombencephalon. Incoming signals trigger the inhibition of sympathetic and the stimulation of parasympathetic structures with accompanying decreasing vasomotor tone, heart rate and contractility. A diagnosis of a carotid sinus hypersensitivity syndrome is established when, during appropriately performed carotid sinus massage [38, 71,224,231,256,311] without administration of conduction-inhibiting drugs, asystole of ≥3 s (cardioinhibitory response), a decline in blood pressure of ≥50 mmHg (vasodepressor response) or both (mixed type) occurs. Contraindications must be observed [153]. Carotid sinus massage is recommended in patients with syncope aged >40 years and where the diagnostic work-up has not yielded an underlying cause [33].

Situational syncope is associated with a sudden loss of voluntary muscle tone and consciousness triggered by a specific prior event. Particular examples of the manifold possible trigger events are: defecation, micturition, coughing, swallowing, pain, emotional upset or physical exercise. Underlying pathophysiological mechanisms are varied, possible causes are due to abnormalities of reflex arcs of the autonomic nervous system as well as central neurotransmitter imbalances.

Chronic vasodilator therapy enhances susceptibility to all three types of neurally mediated reflex syncope. Discontinuation of medication (class I) and maintenance of sufficient intravascular volume (class II) are accepted recommendations.

1.2.3.2 Category 2: Cardiac syncope

The pathophysiology of cardiac syncope is varied and can be classified into three broad categories (Table 1).

The most significant predictor for mortality in syncopal patients is the presence of a structural heart disease [145,208].

Patients with an abnormal 12 lead ECG have an increased 1-year mortality risk [145,208]. Cardiac syncope is associated with a higher mortality rate and an increased sudden cardiac death risk [73,146,178,207].

In patients with structural heart disease the occurrence of syncope is associated with a worse prognosis, regardless of its etiology [145]. The development of syncope in a patient with aortic stenosis without cardiac valve replacement is associated with an estimated two year survival [275].

A history of syncope, at the time of diagnosis with hypertrophic cardiomyopathy, together with a family history of sudden cardiac death, severe dyspnoea and young age are the most significant predictors of sudden cardiac death in this patient subgroup [212].

Table 1 Causes of cardiac syncope (regardless of their etiology, e.g. ischemic, hypertensive, metabolic, inflammatory, myocardial-infiltrative, etc.)

Arrhythmic *bradycardic* • Sinus node and AV-node dysfunctions • Primary asystole *tachycardic* • Paroxysmal supraventricular and ventricular tachycardias • Congenital conduction system diseases (e.g. Brugada syndrome, Romano-Ward syndrome, arrhythmogenic right ventricular dysplasia) and acquired conduction system diseases (e.g. drug-induced long QT syndrome, or ischemic or caused by electrolyte imbalance). • Cardiac arrhythmias caused by pacemaker or defibrillator malfunction
Obstructive • Aortic stenosis • HOCM • Pulmonary embolism • Atrial myxoma • Pericardial disease/tamponade and extracardial compression
Regurgitative • Mitral regurgitation • Aortic regurgitation

Patients with arrhythmogenic right ventricular dysplasia have a similarly adverse prognosis if syncope occurs [69]. Syncope during exercise is an alarming symptom, as opposed to the benign prognosis of patients with post-exercise syncopal events.

There are few possible causes of sudden cardiac death in patients aged ≥35 years, whereas there are many in the patient group aged ≤35 years. While the older group is clearly dominated by coronary heart disease, in younger patients the dominant conditions are hypertropic cardiomyopathy, coronary abnormalities, aortic aneurysms, myocarditis and arrhythmogenic right ventricular dysplasia [205,206,262]. The most frequently encountered cause of syncope in patients after myocardial infarction and intraventricular block is ventricular tachycardia [32]. In this context a QRS-duration of >0.16 s has been shown to be an independent predictor of sudden cardiac death. An invasive electrophysiological work-up is recommended for every patient affected by a combination of myocardial infarction, syncope and intraventricular block [32].

Determination of JTc-time might be useful since findings indicate a high sensitivity of this parameter for the diagnosis of abnormal ventricular repolarization and autonomic cardiac dysfunction.

1.2.3.3 Category 3: Orthostatic syncope

Orthostatic syncope must be differentiated from orthostatic hypotension. The latter is associated with an immediate symptomatic reaction in response to adopting the upright position after lying supine or sitting, the underlying mechanism being cerebral hypoperfusion due to a transiently insufficient compensatory adjustment. Orthostatic intolerance, or orthostatic hypotension, is defined as a decrease in systolic blood pressure of ≥20 mmHg or in diastolic blood pressure of ≥10 mmHg upon standing and within three minutes after the change of posture. It represents a separate clinical manifestation [31].

Orthostatic syncope is defined as a lack of compensatory adjustment due to withdrawal of sympathetic tone. Both orthostatic intolerance and orthostatic syncope are aggravated by all types of volume depletion, hemorrhage or hypovolemia.

Primary or secondary diseases of the autonomic nervous system can be accompanied by an impaired or failed response to hemodynamic changes. Primary autonomic failure syndromes comprise pure autonomic failure with an absence of other neurological diseases, the Shy-Drager syndrome, striatonigral and olivopontocerebellar degeneration [312] and Parkinson's disease. Secondary autonomic failure syndromes are caused by various diseases [13], such as diabetes mellitus, alcohol abuse, kidney or liver disorder. Several drugs can induce autonomic failure, especially antihistamines, tricyclic antidepressants, phenothiazines, MAO-inhibitors and levodopa.

1.2.3.4 Category 4: Subclavian steal syndrome as a cause of syncope

Proximal stenosis, or an obstruction of the subclavian artery, results in retrograde blood flow in the ipsilateral vertebral artery in favor of the equilateral arm. This can cause intermittent hypoperfusion of the brain stem especially during strenuous exercise of the arm when there is a concomitant increased oxygen demand. As a consequence, symptoms can arise such as vertigo, loss of consciousness with spontaneous recovery, and temporary loss of voluntary muscle tone. More frequent though are symptoms like ophthalmophlegia accompanied by diplopia, speech disorders, dysphagia or weakness of the arm muscles, about which detailed information must be obtained from the patient.

1.2.3.5 Differentiation from "non-syncopal" conditions

Various conditions resemble syncope in two different ways: In the first, actual loss of consciousness occurs, but is caused by metabolic disorders (e.g. hypoglycemia), cerebral apoplexy, cerebral hemorrhage, asphyxia, trauma, hyperventilation resulting in hypocapnia, by epilepsy or regionally limited cerebral perfusion (vertebro-basilar transient ischemic attacks). In others, namely somatic psychogenic disorders such as anxiety disorders, hysteria or cataplexy, consciousness is only apparently lost. In these two groups there is either no spontaneous, rapid and complete recovery, or the loss of consciousness is not caused by cerebral hypoperfusion, and therefore do not match the definition of syncope.

Diagnostic and economic considerations warrant the differentiation of syncope from non-syncopal conditions, so that an adequate diagnosis can be obtained, appropriate treatment strategies assessed, and those patients, whose further therapeutic measures do not warrant hospitalization, can be identified. In this respect, as in the prognostically important differentiation of syncopes caused by structural heart diseases from other types of syncope, the use of diagnostic parameters and predefined questionnaires is an important investigative tool.

1.2.3.5.1 Neurological diseases

This comprises disorders that can cause real syncopes or similar conditions that can be accompanied by falls and impaired consciousness, followed by a more or less spontaneous recovery.

a) Epilepsy

Unlike in the case of syncope there is usually no prompt recovery from the loss of consciousness. Epilepsy is often followed by a phase of impaired vigilance, which may be variable in duration. It is also defined by the absence of syncope-inducing cerebral hypoperfusion, loss of consciousness is rare.

In discriminating between them questioning eye-witnesses and patients is helpful. There are usually also a number of symptoms pointing towards one or the other entity [131], which must be assessed through careful history-taking. The immense value of detailed questionnaires cannot be over emphasized.

Clinically, it may be difficult to differentiate seizures from so-called convulsive syncope. However, epileptic clonic movements of the extremities are usually synchronized and tonic extensions frequent, while asynchronous movements of limbs of short duration indicate a syncopal attack. Tongue biting and residual muscle pains point to epilepsy.

b) Transient-ischemic attacks (TIA)

Loss of consciousness is rarely caused by TIAs in the vertebro-basilar circulation, while other symptoms such as vertigo, visual disturbances are observed more frequently [33]. If adhering to the restricted definition of syncope TIAs should be considered among the non-syncopal conditions.

"Drop-attack" is a term that is not clearly defined regarding its etiology and clinical manifestation, but sometimes considered as a TIA in the vertebro-basilar circulation. Loss of consciousness is not an obligatory feature.

c) Migraine

An association between migraine and syncope has been described [204,210], but the actual relationship is not known and has not been studied in detail. The frequency of both disorders suggests that any association may be purely coincidence.

d) Cataplexy

A sudden loss of muscle tone triggered by emotions, either as an independent condition or as part of narcolepsy. The absence of loss of consciousness is the most important feature in distinguishing it from syncope.

1.2.3.5.2 Psychiatric diseases

Linzer has confirmed [183] that 24% of patients with a suspected diagnosis of syncope also had a psychiatric diagnosis. Another study showed a 35% prevalence of psychiatric disorders [140], of which the most common are anxiety and panic disorders and major depression. Hyperventilation can cause a condition resembling syncope. Tilt table examinations may trigger symptoms resembling syncope, but normal hemodynamic response enables the identification of its psychiatric origin.

1.2.3.5.3 Postural orthostatic tachycardia syndrome (POTS)

A diagnosis of POTS can be made by means of tilt table testing [113]:

1. An increase in heart rate of at least 30 bpm within 10 minutes of assuming the upright position when compared to baseline supine values
2. Heart rate ≥120 bpm
3. Stable blood pressure, i.e. no fall of systolic blood pressure of >20 mmHg or drop of diastolic blood pressure of >10 mmHg
4. Symptoms of orthostatic intolerance

Unlike in orthostatic intolerance, there is no decrease of blood pressure, and unlike in syncope there is no loss of consciousness. Hypotension or bradycardia are not symptoms of postural orthostatic tachycardia syndrome. The latter can correctly be defined as an orthostatic reaction with significant tachycardia, the symptoms resemble those of an extended presyncopal phase.

In 80% of cases, POTS affects female patients of predominantly young age [80,188]. Symptomatic features comprise intolerance to prolonged standing with feelings of emptiness, weakness, tremulousness, palpitations, shaky legs and the need to assume a sitting or supine position.

Syncope

Neurally mediated reflex syncope
- Vasovagal syncope
- Carotid sinus hypersensitivity
- Situational syncope

Cardiac syncope
- Obstruction
(e.g. aortic stenosis, HOCM, pulmonary embolism, atrial myxoma, pericardial tamponade)
- Insufficiency
(e.g. aortic/mitral valve insufficiency)
- Arrhythmia → bradycardia, → tachycardia

Orthostatic syncope
- Fluid depletion, hemorrhage
- Primary autonomic failure
(e.g. pure autonomic failure, multiple system atrophy, Parkinson's disease)
- Secondary autonomic failure
(e.g. in the course of diabetes mellitus, alcohol abuse, kidney and liver disorders, drug-induced)

Vascular steal syndromes

Non-syncopal conditions

Neurological diseases
- Epilepsy
- Vertebro-basilar TIA
- Migraine
- Cataplexy

Psychogenic
- Hyperventilation
- Anxiety/panic disorders
- Depression

Postural orthostatic tachycardia syndrome

Figure 2 Classification of syncope, differentiation from non-syncopal conditions

POTS seems to be caused by a dysfunctional sympathetic-mediated vasoconstriction of the peripheral vessels, possibly due to increased norepinephrine release [137] with a compensatory excessive heart rate.

A central pathophysiological feature is the reduced peripheral vasoconstriction, leading to pooling of blood in the lower limbs and subsequent diminished central blood volume with a consistent baroreceptor reflex, thus causing considerable chronotropic exertion.

According to Diehl [80] this increased strain on the heart may provoke anxiety-triggered hyperventilation in susceptible patients, with hypocapnia-caused cerebral vasoconstriction, which is responsible for the subjective symptoms.

The therapeutic approach is similar to that of vasovagal syncope, consisting of sufficient fluid intake and psychosomatically oriented training aimed at easing tension.

1.2.4 Epidemiology

Syncope accounts for 1 to 6% of general hospital admissions and for 3 to 5% of emergency room visits [73,217,292]. 16 to 35% of patients have syncope-related falls with injuries that need medical attention [73,146]. According to conservative estimations at least 3% of the population can be expected to experience a syncopal attack within an observation period of 25 years [282]. The incidence is 6.2 per 1000 person-years [296]. Campell [51] maintains that among the elderly 10% of all falls are attributable to syncope, with the estimated medical treatment costs averaging 700 million dollars per year. Faced with the serious but often underestimated influence of the disease, Great Britain has addressed the problem by initiating government lead initiatives [314].

1.2.5 Mortality

The most significant prognostic marker for syncope-related mortality is the presence of structural heart disease. The 1-year mortality in patients with cardiac syncope ranges between 18 and 33%, compared with a 6% mortality in patients with unexplained syncope, or 0 to 12% in syncope patients with non-cardiac causes [73,141,142,207,292]. 1-year incidence of sudden death was 24% in patients of the first group compared with 3 to 4% in the second group. A particularly high risk group of patients are those suffering from congenital heart failure with a low left ventricular ejection fraction and syncope, where there is a 45% risk of sudden cardiac death at 1 year, compared to the control group of patients with congenital heart failure without syncope, whose risk was 12% [214]. The presence of structural heart disease is the most important prognostic marker of mortality, and patients with impaired left ventricular function have the worst prognosis [309].

In contrast to the high mortality associated with the presence of structural heart disease the following subgroups of patients who have an excellent prognosis [33] can be identified within the total range of patients:

1. Young, healthy patients without cardiac disease and normal resting 12 lead ECG [208]
2. Patients with neurally mediated reflex syncopes [147]
3. Patients with orthostatic hypotension in the absence of serious co-morbidity
4. Patients with syncopes of unknown origin without serious injuries [73,141,142,269,292]

1.2.6 Recurrences

About 35% of patients experience another syncopal episode, with 82% occurring within the first year [146,142]. Recurrent syncopes are not associated with a higher risk of mortality, but may lead to an impaired quality of life.

1.2.7 Diagnosis

In the setting of suspected syncope it is very important to be able to answer two questions: First, was the event an actual syncopal attack fulfilling the definition or was it a non-syncopal condition; second, if syncope is diagnosed, is it related to cardiac disease or not?

In order to ascertain the exact circumstances of a suspected syncope situation it is important to obtain a detailed medical history. In this context bystander observations can be helpful. Questionnaires can provide decisive information as to the presence or absence of syncope while at the same time suggesting a possible etiology. The use of this diagnostic tool is of considerable importance as the undirected use of medical history together with physical examination yields a diagnostic accuracy of only 45% [185].

The analysis of a questionnaire should lead to specific diagnostic parameters [54, 66, 67], with the goal being to initiate a symptom-related diagnostic work-up without, however, initiating a diagnostically and economically ineffective use of all available diagnostic tools.

Even an abnormal response to one single test, e.g. a syncopal attack during tilt table testing, the occurrence of asystole caused by carotid sinus stimulation or of a symptomatic bradycardia during Holter monitoring, does – theoretically – not prove the causal relationship to syncope, even if in practice it is accepted as such [15]. A limiting factor in the diagnosis of syncope is the absence of parallel blood pressure recordings if external or implantable loop-recorders are used. At the moment such devices offering combined recordings are being developed.

Basic evaluation comprises a detailed medical history, physical examination, 12-lead ECG, blood pressure measurement in both arms, measurement of blood-glucose and, if applicable, the administration of a defined questionnaire.

The detailed medical history should include the following features: prescribed drugs, background or past disorders like epilepsy, cardiac or pulmonary diseases, embolisms, cerebral apoplexy, psychiatric disorders, migraine, a detailed family history including questions about similar symptoms or sudden cardiac death, Parkinson's disease, narcolepsy or diabetes. Questions about past operations, especially regarding the digestive system, are useful to suggest a likelihood of dumping syndrome.

Physical examination should include auscultation for cardiac murmurs whilst supine and during a change of position. Other important diagnostic markers are inflow congestion, cyanosis, signs of heart failure as well as tongue biting, signs of volume depletion or hemorrhage, pallor, fetor or paresis. Trigeminal trigger zones and pulse state are features of the symptom-oriented examination.

If the initial evaluation has yielded clear indications of a possible etiology, individual diagnostic procedures should be performed, e.g. an immediate echocardiography in case of suspected heart valve disease, immediate duplex ultrasonography in the case of differences in blood pressure in the two arms. In the case of suspected cardiac ischemia its immediate exclusion or instantaneous coronary angiography is warranted.

If the initial evaluation does not yield any suggestive results, the next step should be the review of the specific questionnaire; its questions should correspond to, and be suggestive of, specific causes. After its analysis, each set of possible causes should be evaluated, starting with the potentially most dangerous disorder. If the following diagnostic procedure establishes a definite diagnosis, there will be no need for diagnostic evaluations in other fields. If the procedure yields no results, then a reappraisal of the patient work-up should follow, together with further individual assessment. No further diagnostic evaluations are recommended, if the following conditions are fulfilled [33]:

a) Probable benign character of syncope (no risk occupation [pilot, bus operator or physician], rare occurrence [$\leq 1\times$/year], age <35 years, no cardiac disease, no serious injuries)
b) Probability of vasovagal syncope
c) Orthostatic hypotension

According to the guidelines of the European Society of Cardiology [33,34] the initial evaluation yields a certain diagnosis in the following cases:

- Vasovagal syncope: occurrence of typical trigger situations like prolonged standing or emotional or painful stimuli

- Situational syncope: after defecation, micturition, coughing or swallowing
- Orthostatic syncope: documented fall in systolic blood pressure of >20 mmHg or to <90 mmHg
- Syncope due to cardiac ischemia with indicative symptoms, typical ECG results and/or biomarkers
- Arrhythmogenic syncope if a resting-ECG yields the following abnormalities:
  - Sinus bradycardia <40 bpm or intermittent sino-atrial block with sinus arrest >3 s,
  - 3rd degree AV-block and Mobitz II 2nd degree
  - Intermittent complete left or right bundle branch block
  - Rapid supraventricular or ventricular tachycardia
  - Pacemaker malfunction

1.2.7.1 Diagnostic tools

Depending upon the outcome of the initial evaluation which includes a careful medical history or the evaluation of a "syncope questionnaire", further diagnostic steps should be taken in a target-oriented and strategic manner [15] as the use of only a single diagnostic tool has a low success rate in identifying causes of syncope.

According to Kapoor [43] laboratory tests yield results of diagnostic importance only in 2 to 3% of all cases, echocardiography is diagnostically useful in 5 to 10% of all patients, computed tomography in 4% of patients, EEG in 2% of all cases, prolonged ECG monitoring in 4%. Even an extension of Holter monitoring to 72 hours does not improve accuracy for diagnosing syncope. The use of so-called "loop recorders", which enable patients to transmit telemetric ECG recordings, confirms an arrhythmic cause of syncope in 8 to 20% [48,184]. The symptom arrhythmia correlation using implantable loop recorders seems to be improved [163].

All this advocates the selective and algorithm-controlled use of diagnostic procedures including the analysis of questionnaires. Diagnostic and economic considerations dispute the usefulness of diagnostic procedures following the "water can principle". Considering the frequency of a vasovagal etiology of syncope, it could be suggested that tilt table testing be the primary diagnostic device which may open the way for diagnostic evaluation on an outpatient basis. Kapoor [143] has outlined possible indications for in-hospital assessment.

In the situation where there is evidence of a structural heart origin and after exclusion of acute cardiac ischemia then transthoracic echocardiography is recommended, under some circumstances (aortic disorders, intracardiac tumors and thromboembolisms) accompanied by transesophageal imaging. If echocardiography does not reveal the underlying disturbance, first an exercise test should be performed to detect the presence of coronary heart disease. Depending upon the results, invasive evaluation by means of coronary angiography is recommended.

Other diagnostic tools to identify causes of syncope, or to identify patients with possible risks, are Holter monitoring including heart rate variability, ventricular after depolarizations, T wave alternans, external or implantable event recorders [99,162,161,227], pharmacological provocation testing, invasive electrophysiologic assessments [99] and right ventricular catheterization.

If the basic evaluation is suggestive of carotid sinus hypersensitivity, it should be followed immediately by carotid sinus massage according to the protocols proposed by Brignole [42] and Parry [256]. Carotid sinus massage is the recommended procedure for patients aged >40 years where initial evaluation has not yielded underlying causes [33].

The immediate occurrence of symptoms upon changes of posture can be detected by means of the Schellong test and subsequently classified as orthostatic intolerance.

Should symptoms arise after straining one or both arms, duplex ultrasonography should be performed to identify a subclavian steal phenomenon. Duplex ultrasonography is also the method of choice if symptoms like speech disorders or diplopia prior to loss of consciousness occur, since these are indicative of transient ischemic attacks in the brain stem. If these diagnostic procedures produce new information, other applicable tools are angiography, computed tomography and magnetic resonance imaging.

If the medical history and/or the syncope questionnaire suggest psychiatric causes, a specialist colleague should be included in the patient treatment, as well as in the case of the interdisciplinary planning of further diagnostic measures and treatment strategies for possible epilepsy. Another situation where an interdisciplinary therapeutic approach is recommended is loss of consciousness triggered by severe facial pain, indicating glossopharyngeal or trigeminal neuralgia; or the occurrence of reproducible postprandial syncope, which – if there is a history of subtotal or complete gastrectomy – might point towards a dumping syndrome.

Where findings pointing towards vasovagal or situational syncope, tilt table testing is the investigation of choice, as well as being a supplementary diagnostic tool if the initial evaluation does not yield any specific results. A positive response to tilt table testing renders further diagnostic measures obsolete if typical clinical features can be observed.

1.2.7.2 Tilt table testing

On moving from a supine to an upright posture there is a gravitational shift of 300–800 ml of blood to the venous capacitance system within the first 10 s of standing, followed by a decrease in cardiac filling pressure and in stroke volume.

In addition, a reduction of intravascular volume, due to increased capillary transmural pressure, and filtration of protein-free fluid into the interstitial spaces can be observed.

In order to maintain arterial blood pressure there is a compensatory increase in heart rate, which, however, is insufficient on its own. The key adjustment mechanism is a vasoconstriction of the musculoskeletal, visceral and renal arteries, a mechanism mediated exclusively by the automatic nervous system with its pressor receptors, afferent and efferent pathways.

During prolonged standing, additional mechanisms like the renin-angiotensin-aldosterone system are activated to maintain a sufficient level of arterial organ perfusion.

Failure of compensatory mechanisms is thought to be the cause of vasovagal syncope and represents the basis for using tilt table testing.

1.2.7.2.1 Indications

A consensus document by the European Society of Cardiology [33] outlines several current indications for tilt table testing (Table 2), and similar indications can be found in a paper published by the German Society of Cardiology [77]. Both of these guidelines do not consider the potential future developments in tilt table testing when combined with non-invasive monitoring.

Over time the diagnostic application of tilt table testing has been considerably extended.

A classical indication is the assessment of recurrent syncope, presyncope, or single syncopal episodes in high risk patients (pilots, bus operators, scaffolders). Recommendations for tilt table testing have also been extended to include older patients with unexplained falls [123], diagnosis and differentiation of convulsive syncopal episodes [108,123,333] and epilepsy, especially if the latter has proved re-

Table 2 Indications advocating tilt table testing [33]

Class I • In the case of unexplained single episodes of syncope in high risk patients, or recurrent syncope in patients without structural heart disease, or in patients with structural heart disease after cardiac causes have been excluded. • When it is of value to demonstrate susceptibility to vasovagal syncope to the patient.
Class II • When a classification into the diagnostic category of vasovagal syncope might alter the therapeutic approach. • For evaluating patients with recurrent unexplained falls. • For diagnosing patients with recurrent presyncope and dizziness.
Class III • Therapeutic review • Assessment of a single episode when potential high risk features are absent. • In the case of unmistakable vasovagal features when the respective diagnosis would not alter treatment.

sistant to treatment, as well as the differentiation from orthostatic hypotension [64], postural orthostatic tachycardia syndrome [116], psychogenic and hyperventilation "syncopes" [232,272] and carotid sinus hypersensitivity [130,152,211].

Tilt table testing is also a potential tool for the evaluation of recurrent vertigo with or without indications of central dysautonomic or peripheral neuropathic disorders.

Based upon these classical indications the passive orthostatic evaluation, combined with other non-invasive evaluation procedures may be extended to other conditions.

Testing of cardiovascular autonomic function, identification of patients with high risk profiles after myocardial infarction, development of new pharmacological and non-pharmacological therapeutic approaches and optimization of pacemaker and defibrillator therapies are some of its potential uses. In addition there exists indicative evidence of possible uses in the diagnosis of chronic fatigue syndrome or sudden infant death [121,114].

Potential and future uses surpass by far the classical recommendations (Table 2). There is, however currently, no scientific consensus as to the extent of their value [33,77].

1.2.7.2.2 Contraindications

Kenny [153] states that there are no absolute contraindications to the use of tilt table testing because of the low rate of complications. Relative contraindications may be in severe left ventricular outflow obstruction, serious mitral stenosis, as well as significant circulation-related cardiac or cerebrovascular stenosis. Administration of isoprotenerol for drug provocation may trigger dangerous arrhythmias, so it is contraindicated in susceptible patients.

1.2.7.2.3 Protocol

General conditions for performing tilt table testing can be found in Table 3.

Tilt table testing protocols are varied, not only in respect of the equipment used, but particularly regarding time, duration of supine and upright phases, tilt angle and the use of provocative agents.

Table 3 Recommendations for tilt table testing

- Patients should be well informed and should fast for at least 2 hours before the test, preferably overnight.
- Room should be quiet and with the right temperature.
- Continuous beat-to-beat monitoring of blood pressure and heart rate, as well as constant ECG monitoring.
- Immediately available medical staff.
- Immediately available resuscitation team and equipment.
- Supine position for 5 minutes before tilting, and for at least 20 minutes if vascular cannulation is employed.
- Tilt table of the foot-board support type, angles should be able to be set quickly as well as slowly and smoothly.
- Multiple tests should be performed preferably at the same time of day.
- Tilt angle of 60–70°.
- For drug provocation with isoprotenerol, a constant infusion rate from 1–3 µg/min in order to increase average heart rate 20–25% over baseline, or sublingual administration of 400 µg nitroglycerin.

a) Tilt angle

In the first publication advocating the use of tilt table testing, Kenny [151] used a tilt angle of 60° with a tilt duration of 60 minutes. In 1991, Fitzpatrick [90] demonstrated that a tilt angle of <60° was associated with a lower rate of positive responses. The mean time to positive responses was 24 minutes. The method which is today known as the Westminster protocol proposes settings of 60° over 45 minutes. Later various modified protocols have been used with tilt angles between 20° and 90° and tilt duration of 2–60 minutes [156].

Established protocols use tilt angles between 60° and 80° and tilt duration varies from 40–60 minutes [3,9,17,29,50,89,118,120, 151,153,178,266,303,310]. Tilt angles below 60° are known to reduce sensitivity, whereas angles of more than 80° have an adverse effect on the specificity of the result [147,156,233]. The precise angle when ranging between 60° and 90° seems to be of less importance [156].

Most studies use a tilt angle of 60° or 70°. Studies without drug provocation show a specificity in the order of 90% [16].

b) Tilt duration
Unlike the choice of tilt angle, the duration of passive tilt phase appears to have greater influence. To be able to differentiate orthostatic hypotension from orthostatic syncope, the upright tilt phase should be longer than 10 minutes [156].

Various different studies have reported using an upright phase duration between 10 and 60 minutes [3,9,17,29,50,89,118,120, 151,178,266,303,310]. Most, however, advocate a longer duration of the un-medicated phase, mostly 45 minutes, followed by drug provocation if the test has so far yielded no positive response.

Test phases with 30–45 minutes of a first drug-free postural phase and tilt angles between 60 and 80° and without drug challenge are the ones most frequently encountered. Fitzpatrick [90] proposed that the passive phase of tilting be determined according to the mean duration to syncope ±2 standard deviations, resulting in a passive phase of about 45 minutes.

A "shortened" protocol including sublingual nitroglycerin provocation (10 minutes of supine pre-tilt phase, a passive phase of 20 minutes at 60°, then, if necessary, challenge with 400 µg nitroglycerin sublingually, followed by another upright phase of 20 minutes) is favored over more time-intensive protocols with the same level of specificity and sensitivity [75].

The mean duration to syncope varies according to different studies and ranges between 22 and 24 minutes [90,147] at 60° and around 7 minutes at 70° [297].

c) Drug challenge
In 1989, Almquist [9] and Waxman [323] were the first to include a drug challenge in tilt table testing, with the administration of isoprotenerol to provoke syncope, assuming that this triggers an aggravated cardiac response with potential excessive stimulation of myocardial C-fibers and a subsequent withdrawal of sympathetic tone with bradycardia/asystole and/or hypotension. This maneuver yielded a higher rate of positive responses. The use of isoprotenerol has also been modified in several instances [144,221,233],

with reported specificity rates ranging between 45% [144] and 93% [233].

In 1994, Raviele [270] proposed intravenous – and later sublingual – administration of nitroglycerin for drug challenge purposes, showing an increased specificity of 94%. Comparative studies of both substances showed similar specificity but higher tolerance of sublingually administered nitroglycerin.

The duration of the un-medicated phase before drug challenge is still a controversial issue. A comparison between 5 and 45 minutes showed that the longer un-medicated phases yielded a higher rate of positive responses [14]. A duration of 20 minutes [75,94,235], however, does not seem to be inferior to a duration of 45 minutes [14,94].

The analysis of heart rate variability over 5 minutes in supine position before tilting may yield valuable information regarding the recommendable choice of provocative drugs. In the study of Nino et al. [237] in patients, who had shown positive responses after nitroglycerin challenge but had stayed asymptomatic when challenged with isoprotenerol and vice versa, there were different profiles of heart rate variability, which was analyzed on the basis of the sympatho-vagal balance (LF/HF-ratio). In patients with vasovagal syncope challenged by nitroglycerin administration a significantly lower ratio was observed, compared with the group of patients with isoprotenerol-induced syncope. The authors postulate the presence of vagotony in the group which showed positive responses to nitroglycerin challenge, and the presence of exaggerated sympathetic strain in the latter group. This indicates that the choice of the appropriate provocative agent might be made even before the orthostatic stress phase.

Studies suggest that invasive measurement of arterial blood pressure may cause a significantly higher incidence of syncope being in response to the venous cannulation process itself [301]. If intra-arterial techniques are favored over non-invasive continuous measurement of blood pressure by means of finger-plethysmography, more time should be allowed for equilibration.

Findings of these studies have been included in international [16,33] and national [77] recommendations for performing tilt table tests. Keeping in mind the existence of department-specific structures and strategies, no standard-protocol can be proposed that is equally suited to all users.

1.2.7.2.4 Reproducibility

The reproducibility of tilt table tests has been studied in several instances [55,74,97]. These have shown that the overall reproducibility of an initial negative response ranges between 85 to 94%, and is thus higher than the reproducibility of an initial positive response (31 to 91%). However, 50% of all patients with a baseline positive test show subsequent negative reactions when receiving treatment or placebo [222,228,264].

Chen [55] observed a test response correspondence of 87% in two rapidly successive tests (within 1 hour) in 23 patients. The group with an initial positive response showed a reduced correspondence rate, additionally, 3 out of 15 patients had a positive response only during the initial test. In contrast, all initially negative patients also showed negative responses in the subsequent test.

Longer intervals between the two tests (1–7 days [266] up to 4 years [259]) showed similar rates of reproducibility, i.e. 62 to 90% [30,122,259,266].

Overall reproducibility ranges are between 65 and 85% and is independent of the chosen intervals between tests. Initial negative responses are rarely followed by positive ones. However, because of varied measurement protocols, reproducibility data is not fully comparable.

1.2.7.2.5 Special issues in evaluating pediatric or elderly patients

Tilt table tests are considered feasible for children aged >6 years [119,151,178,262,274]. Compared with the number of studies involving adult patients, there is less available information about the use of tilt table testing in children. In contrast to measurement techniques in adults, blood pressure measurement in children should be restricted to non-invasive methods. As in the case of adult patients, a typical clinical diagnosis of vasovagal syncope in correlation with otherwise normal findings of the initial evaluation can render tilt table testing unnecessary. It should be noted that a child's lower center of gravity is associated with lower orthostatic stress, which may make it necessary to use a longer test duration or a steeper tilt angle.

In most studies, however, the usual examination protocols were applicable to children [16,46,107,126,127,147,219,328]. Positive responses tend to occur earlier and the mixed response type, defined according to the VASIS-classification, is the dominant one.

Opinions differ as to the validity of the gained parameters. It is not generally possible to measure a child's smaller stroke volume accurately by means of impedance cardiography, and in addition exaggerated ventilation is an influence in pediatric patients [70]. The rate of false measurements can be reduced by modified electrodes and improved measuring methods [95,96].

It is difficult to evaluate older patients. In view of the great range of secondary disorders, even a positive tilt response cannot exclude an underlying disorder actually causing the symptoms. Cardiovascular medication warrants special attention.

1.2.7.2.6 Interpretation of tilt table test results

Examinations where the patient is asymptomatic should be considered negative results. Drug-associated hypotension after nitroglycerin challenge (exaggerated response) [265,270] must also be differentiated from vasodepressor syncope.

According to Kenny [153], test results can be defined as positive when the occurring symptoms correspond to those typically known to the patient and if associated with hypotension, bradycardia (relative or absolute) or both. Isolated reduction of blood pressure and heart rate with minor or no symptoms does not justify a diagnosis of vasovagal syncope.

In the situation of a positive response, Sutton [306] proposed a classification system in 1992, which is today known as the VASIS classification (Table 7) that is based on the hemodynamic patterns before and during syncope.

Its distinguishing features are only applicable if syncope occurs, which is why the moment of tilt termination is important. The ideal moment is precisely when loss of consciousness occurs. Premature interruption underestimates and delayed interruption overestimates the cardioinhibitory response and exposes the patient to prolonged loss of consciousness.

Various studies [34,112,265,270] have analyzed the presyncopal phase, identifying different patterns [33]. The derived classification is presented in Table 8.

Two different reaction patterns are the most frequently encountered. The typical pattern of the so-called "classic" type consists of an initial phase of complete adaptation to the upright position with stable blood pressure and heart rate, thus suggesting normal baroreflex function, until the onset of the vasovagal reaction. This hemodynamic reaction is prevalent in young, and otherwise healthy patients, with a long history of recurrent syncopal episodes starting in very young age. They are assumed to be caused by a hypersensitive autonomic system that over-responds to changed hemodynamic demands.

The other pattern, the so-called "dysautonomic" type, is characterized by an inability to adapt to the postural change. The initial increase in heart rate is insufficient or altogether absent, during the presyncopal phase a progressive fall in blood pressure and heart rate occurs until the onset of syncope. While an exaggerated reaction can be observed in the classic pattern, the latter is characterized by a slow or absent reaction to changed hemodynamic demands. Those patients are usually older and have significant co-morbidities, they have a short history of syncopal episodes with few recurrences. Tilt table testing can assist in distinguishing those patterns.

1.2.7.2.7 Limitations and complications

Tilt table testing is a safe procedure with few complications. Syncope with or without asystole can be interrupted simply by returning the patient to supine position. Life-threatening arrhythmias have only been reported in patients suffering from coronary heart disease or the sick sinus syndrome after administration of isoprotenerol

[100,175]. No complications have been reported associated with the use of nitroglycerin, but side-effects like vertigo, headache and palpitations are frequent. On account of the mentioned negative responses in initially positively responding patients without prior pharmacological treatment, or after placebo treatment, the use of tilt table testing for the evaluation of treatment is limited. Therapeutic success should be interpreted cautiously [222,228]. As opposed to its diagnostic value, tilt table testing is not an accepted method for therapeutic control.

1.2.8 Therapy of neurally mediated reflex syncope

Because of the major differences in morbidity pattern and mortality risk before considering therapeutic measures it is important to differentiate neurally mediated reflex syncope from cardiac syncope.

Therapy of neurally mediated reflex syncope has two objectives: first, the improvement of quality of life, and second, the reduction of serious consequential damage associated with the condition, especially injuries due to falls and accidents caused by loss of consciousness. The therapeutic goal is more of an alleviating than of remedial character.

Treatment relies mostly on avoiding the trigger event, i.e. prolonged standing, knowledge of the benign nature of the disease in absence of consequential falls or accidents, as well as on the recognition of symptoms possibly preceding a syncopal episode. If symptoms occur, adequate maneuvers to avert the episode are recommended, e.g. changing to supine position or leaving crowded places. Other basic therapeutic strategies include avoiding hypotensive drugs and increasing fluid or salt intake [333] in vasodepressor syncope. A fluid intake of 2.5 liters and sodium intake of 150–250 mmol sodium per day is recommended, as well as 30-minutes exercise three times a week and 10–20 minutes of tilt training per day.

Methodological problems prevent a clear evaluation of therapeutic success. Patients with a baseline positive test often show subsequent negative reactions after placebo treatment [39]. As a result the effectiveness of therapeutic studies without placebo control should be judged with caution. Interestingly, the mere diagnosis of vasovagal syncope reduces its recurrence of symptoms; its natural course, with a tendency towards abatement, is favorable [39,222,234]. There are indications that the demonstration of syncope in a controlled environment assists in an improved recognition of warning symptoms and thus in avoiding high-risk situations [234].

1.2.8.1 Therapy of vasovagal syncope

The therapeutic approaches detailed below reflect the current state of knowledge. Future improvement of measuring methods aimed at identifying the various pathophysiological backgrounds during vasovagal syncopes might assist in developing more individualized therapeutic strategies, whose differential therapeutic approach will intervene in a supportive or inhibitory way in one limb of the autonomic nervous system or will modify central regulatory mechanisms. These future innovations in addition to the already existing and used therapeutic principles are promising.

1.2.8.1.1 Pharmacological therapy

In addition to the previously described basic therapeutic strategies various studies have examined a number of other therapeutic approaches. With the exception of one study involving the use of paroxetine [79], no placebo-controlled trials have been able to show an advantage of pharmacological therapy over placebo [33,194,222, 264], despite the positive results of short-term trials [24,58,92, 121,135,139,177,197,215,230,296,297,313,322]. This is not the case for any of the used drugs (beta-blockers, disopyramide, etilefrine, midodrine, clonidine, fludrocortisone, bronchodilator therapy, scopolamine, ephedride, serotonin reuptake inhibitors, etc.). The possible beneficial effect of paroxetine shall be examined in further trials. Nevertheless and in spite of possible placebo effects, single patient populations can reasonably expect to benefit from pharmacological therapeutic measures. The used substance or, respectively, the substance combination, must definitely be individualized. In addition to conservative measures, younger patients often benefit from low doses of fludrocortisone, from a peripheral alpha-agonist (midodrine) or a central serotonin reuptake inhibitor. On the other hand, older patients' orthostatic symptoms may best be alleviated by discontinuing medication for circulation disorders and by the treatment of underlying co-morbidity (diabetes mellitus, vitamin B_{12} deficiency anemia, renal insufficiency, existence of tumors, etc.). Individualized therapeutic recommendations for each category are not currently available.

1.2.8.1.2 Pacemaker therapy

The therapeutic value of pacemaker therapy is a controversial issue. Head-up tilt laboratory findings have reported that pacing fails to prevent syncope, but prolongs the premonitory warning phase [84,91,260,280,299]. In spite of these findings the studies of the North American vasovagal pacemaker study [62] and the European VASIS trial [305] were able to verify a significant reduction of syncope recurrence in a selected patient population with dual chamber cardiac pacing. The potential weakness [19] of these studies lies in a possible placebo effect due to pacemaker implantation. The European Society of Cardiology recommends that further studies should follow before pacing can become an established therapy. In patients aged >40 years with cardioinhibitory neurally mediated syncope, which either occurs >5 times a year or causes serious injuries, the implantation of a dual chamber cardiac pacemaker is recommended (Class II) [33,34].

In 2003, the first randomized placebo-controlled and double-blind study to demonstrate the therapeutic value of dual chamber cardiac pacing in patients with recurrent syncope [63] was published. It reported no benefit in the group of patients with activated pacing. These findings have subsequently been supported by another randomized placebo-controlled and double-blind study in 2004 [268].

In consideration of these findings it is unlikely that the current restricted recommendation for the use of pacemaker therapy will be extended, except to the cardioinhibitory or mixed types of carotid sinus hypersensitivity, where it is already established.

New algorithms regarding frequency-modified stimulation, based on the analysis of impedance cardiography recordings via the right ventricular electrode, have yielded the first promising results regarding the avoidance of recurrent vasovagal cardioinhibitory syncope [246,247]. But further long-term studies will have to be performed to corroborate the beneficial effect of the therapy.

1.2.8.1.3 Conservative therapy

Domestic tilt training is a simple therapy that has the potential to significantly reduce syncope recurrence and has been labeled as a Class II recommendation [34]. However, despite highly promising short-term results, there are suggestions of a reduced long-term efficacy due to deteriorating patient compliance [2,78,83,271].

Mechanical maneuvers during the phase of impending syncope have been reported to have an alleviating influence [35,164]. These include muscle tension of the extremities, e.g. a tight handgrip for 2 seconds, or tensing movements like multiple leg crossing for 30 seconds. Patients should be informed of these side-effect free therapeutic approaches.

Parry [254] has published a first therapeutic algorithm for treating vasovagal syncope. A confirmed diagnosis of vasovagal syncope is followed by patient education and, if necessary, discontinuation of potentially symptom-provoking drugs. In the case of continuing symptoms and frequently recurrent syncopes, a high grade of suffering or potential danger of accidents, there are two different therapeutic pathways. According to Parry, implantation of a dual chamber cardiac pacemaker is recommended for patients with cardioinhibitory reactions. Should symptoms continue, the patient will be assigned to the second therapeutic pathway. First a 24-hour urine is tested for sodium concentration. If it lies below 170 mmol, a daily dose of 120 mmol of sodium chloride is recommended. When the urine collection yields a higher sodium concentration, or if symptoms continue after administration of sodium, the use of beta-blockers is recommended, and in the case of continuing symptoms, the cascading prescription of fludrocortisone and/or midodrine, possibly followed by paroxetine and further drugs.

1.2.8.2 Therapy of carotid sinus syncope

Therapy is guided by the results of the carotid sinus massage. When there is documented bradycardia and a certain relation between syncope and carotid sinus stimulation, the implantation of a cardiac pacemaker, preferably with dual chamber stimulation, is the therapy of choice [19,38,40,41,44,76,193,213,223]. At present pharmacological treatment is not recommended. There are currently no randomized studies regarding the treatment of the vasodepressor subtype. Positive reactions being enhanced by carotid sinus massage during vasodilator therapy indicate that volume expansion by salt and/or fluid intake may be beneficial.

1.2.8.3 Therapy of situational syncope

When specific trigger events are recognized they should be avoided whenever possible. However, this may be difficult or even impossible, e.g. when emotional upset, pain, defecation, micturition

Table 4 Recommendations for treatment of neurally mediated syncope [34]

Class I
• Explanation about the risk and the benign character of vasovagal syncope.
• Avoidance of trigger events as much as possible or reduction of their magnitude.
• Modification or discontinuation of hypotensive drug medication.
• Cardiac pacing in patients with cardioinhibitory or mixed carotid sinus syndrome.
Class II
• Volume expansion by salt supplementation, an exercise program or head-up sleeping in posture-related syncope.
• Tilt training.
• Isometric leg and arm counter-pressure maneuvers.
• Cardiac pacing in patients with cardioinhibitory vasovagal syncope with a frequency >5 attacks per year or severe physical injury or accidents and age >40.
Class III
• No existing evidence for the efficacy of beta-blockers.

or coughing are triggering agents. In these circumstances sufficient fluid intake, adopting a sitting or supine position or slower changes of posture are recommended measures. Because of the great number of potential triggers there are a wide variety of possible behavioral patterns that patients may adopt in order to avoid loss of consciousness.

Patients with situational syncope often have a positive response to carotid sinus massage and tilt table testing [37], which has potential therapeutic implications, including cardiac pacing. But further study is needed to determine if this is universally the case.

Table 4 outlines the recommendations of the European Society of Cardiology [34].

1.3 Continuous non-invasive blood pressure recording

For many years, exact non-invasive blood pressure monitoring posed serious problems. Since the beginning of the last century efforts have been made to monitor the arterial pulse curve by means of pressure sensors attached to the arterial wall. A major limitation of the method, known as tonometry, was loss of energy of the pulse wave due to the resistance of the vascular wall, thus hindering exact measurements. The method of applanation tonometry attempts to solve this problem by slightly compressing the arterial wall. This technique, however, does not solve the problem of permanent fluctuations of blood pressure amplitude. Penaz [254,257,258] was the first to record those and to use them as a parameter of counter-pressure. By means of a photoelectric sensor the blood flow in the finger was recorded, enabling the regulation of a pneumatic valve which compressed the arterial wall depending upon the blood flow. This procedure leads to a reduction of transmural pressure, and the arterial wall is considered as "unloaded", a state which is maintained by automatic adjustments of the external to the intra-arterial pressure. Wesseling et al. [325] took out a patent on this method in Amsterdam and established it for clinical use (Finapres™ device). It is now known as the "vascular unloading technique" and has subsequently been refined several times for clinical and research use [254].

This device uses an inflatable finger cuff. In the past the more complicated calibration process created substantial problems, as a result its production had been stopped for some time, but new technological advances and the extension of its possible uses has seen its popularity reemerge. Today, continuous self-calibration against oscillometric brachial artery blood pressure measurements enables continuous, non-invasive finger blood pressure monitoring. This method allows for the constant correction of perfusion fluctuations of the finger arteries, which are also subject to regional thermal fluctuations. Their influence may be minimized using the calibration against brachial artery blood pressure measurements. A large body of literature has demonstrated a high degree of conformity between non-invasive and invasive blood measurements [170].

This technique is of crucial importance for the beat-to-beat monitoring of blood pressure, as well as the basis for assessment of spontaneous baroreflex sensitivity and blood pressure variability, which, among other things, reflects the function of the sympathetic system.

1.4 Impedance cardiography

In 1921, variations in thoracic impedance were used for the first time to study cardiac function [11]. Later, methods were developed to determine cardiac output by measuring changes in resistance of a high frequency alternating current field that is applicated to the thorax [240,241,278,326]. In 1966, Kubicek's work laid the basis for the non-invasive assessment of cardiovascular parameters by means of impedance cardiography [165,166,167].

Initial differences in the determined cardiovascular parameters, when compared to measurements derived according to Fick's method and thermodilution techniques, were resolved by refined mathematical formulas that yield an improved correspondence [20,21,300,317] and reproducibility [23].

The impedance cardiogram is recorded by means of electrodes placed on the neck and on the lower thorax. Between the electrodes a constant current of 400 µA with a frequency of 40 kHz is applied to the body and the voltage is derived. A high-ohm internal resistance of the voltage measurement device minimizes current flux through the body. The impedance can be calculated on the basis of Ohm's law. Interfering influences like autoelectric cardiac activity, potential muscle activity, breathing changes, or skin resistance are minimized by means of specially designed electrodes [95] and mathematical procedures using intelligent adaptive digital filtering.

The underlying physiological principle of impedance cardiography is based on the assumption that the thoracic impedance changes in relation to the cardiac cycle, proportionally to the quantity of cardiac output. A systolic shift of blood from the left ventricle into the aorta generates a reduction of electric impedance, since the transferred blood has a lower resistance against the passing current and the epicardium-coated heart, having a high electrical resistance, contracts during systole. Based on parameters of basic impedance and impedance variation during the cardiac cycle, as well as the sex, weight and size of the patient the parameters of cardiovascular function (e.g. stroke volume, cardiac output, contractility, systemic peripheral resistance) can be derived without risk and non-invasively.

By means of the described method, reliable data regarding hemodynamic function is gained without invasive methods like blood withdrawal or right-ventricular catheterization.

Figure 3 Curves of parallel recordings of ECG and impedance cardiography to determine systolic intervals and cardiac output.

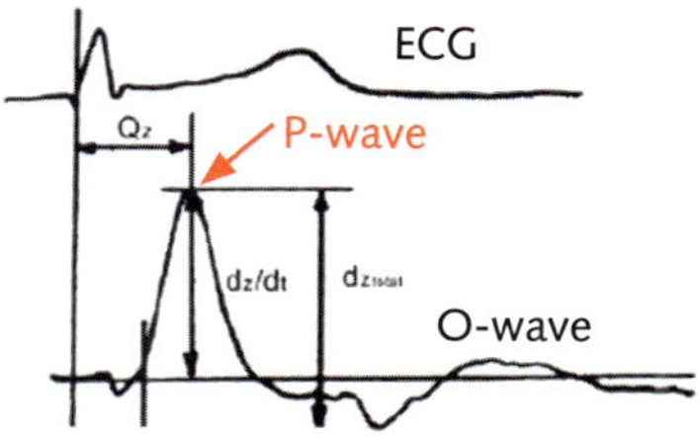

In addition to the analysis of the predetermined contractility parameters, the data available from the impedance signal itself may ultimately provide preliminary non-invasive information (Fig. 3).

The rise in the impedance waveform (P-wave) marks the maximal systolic output. The presence of a left ventricular insufficiency is characterized by reduced amplitude. In the case of a cardiac pacing therapy with right ventricular stimulation or a complete left bundle branch block an interventricular asynchronous contraction can be observed by a biphasic peak. The low rise during diastole (O-wave) marks the opening of the mitral wave. An excessive rise, in distinctive cases even exceeding the P-wave, can be observed in the presence of an increased pressure of the right atrium and of mitral heart defects.

1.5 Further applications of tilt table testing and non-invasive monitoring

The assessment of heart rate variability and baroreflex sensitivity requires continuous ECG- and heart rate monitoring, as well as "beat-to-beat" blood pressure measurement.

To obtain all relevant data regarding the hemodynamic and autonomic functions of an individual during examination, sophisticated mathematical methods and efficient software enable the parallel (but also independent) employment of impedance cardiography, non-invasive blood pressure measurement and continuous ECG-recording during a tilt table test. Modern devices offer a wide range of potential uses that far exceed merely tilt table testing and will be reviewed below.

1.5.1 Baroreflex sensitivity

Baroreflex sensitivity can be defined as the extent of heart rate modification in disproportional relation to change in arterial blood pressure.

A rise in arterial blood pressure generates a lengthening in R-R interval and vice versa.

Afferent pathways, starting in pressor receptors of the larger vessels proximal to the heart, conduct towards the medullary cardiovascular centers and provoke an autonomic efferent regulation of the cardiac chronotropic function by means of a reduced sympathetic nervous system influence.

There are several methods for the measurement of baroreflex sensitivity [252]. The injection of a vasoconstrictive or vasodilative substance causes a change in blood pressure and heart rate without impeding the reflex arc, thus enabling the assessment of baroreflex sensitivity. Other methods include carotid sinus stimulation by massage or controlled compression ("neck chamber"), intermittent orthostasis or the administration of negative pressure in the lower extremities. An important, non-invasive method with high reproducibility is the "sequence method" [85,251,253,254], which consists of un-medicated continuous beat-to-beat monitoring of heart rate and systolic blood pressure. An equivalent change in RR-interval and systolic blood pressure (SBP) for at least three consecutive cardiac cycles is defined as a regulatory event, which is characterized by either a decrease in blood pressure and shortening in RR-interval (–RR/–SBP sequences), a so-called "down-event", or by a rise in blood pressure and lengthening in RR-interval (+RR/+SBP sequences), a so-called "up-event". The number of detected sequences (down-events and up-events) is referred to as the "event count". The baroreflex effectiveness index (BEI) can be defined as the ratio between the total number of detected baroreflex events and the total number of ramp-like changes in blood pressure, regardless of whether the latter are followed by a change in RR-interval or not. The higher the BEI value, the more SBP ramp changes are followed by a change in RR-interval. The approximate normal value of the BEI ranges around 0.58 ± 0.2 [261].

In addition to the baroreflex effectiveness index, there is a second parameter, the so-called "slope", which describes the steepness of the regression line between blood pressure change in mmHg and the RR-interval change in ms, regardless of whether a drop in blood pressure with subsequent RR-interval shortening, or a rise in blood pressure with RR-interval lengthening occurs. For age- and sex-related normal values, see Appendix, Chapter 4.3.

However, only a few studies have exclusively examined the influence of baroreflex sensitivity. Dysfunction can be found in patients with autonomic neuropathies, e.g. diabetic neuropathy, with neurological diseases where areas of the brain stem are involved, with arterial hypotension, or in patients susceptible to vasovagal syncope, etc.

The high predictive value of baroreflex sensitivity for risk stratification after myocardial infarction underlines the correlation between experimental and clinical cardiology and provides insights into the underlying mechanisms of the autonomic cardiac system.

1.5.2 Heart rate variability

In the last three decades various studies have demonstrated the relationship between the function of the autonomic nervous system and cardiovascular mortality [65,179,189,286]. In 1965, Hon and Lee [132] demonstrated the influence of fetal stress on RR-intervals even before a change of heart rate was detectable. Between 1968 and 1981 the existence of hidden physiologic rhythms in RR-interval variability was discovered. In 1977, Wolf [327] was the first to detect the correlation between reduced heart rate variability and an increased risk in patients after a myocardial infarction. Since then, the procedure has been refined on multiple occasions [6,19] and has emerged as a clear-cut independent predictor of mortality after a myocardial infarction [25,157,200].

At present there are various parameters of heart rate variability. One definition describes it as the difference between the shortest and the longest RR-intervals within a defined test period.

Heart rate variability is classically obtained during prolonged ECG monitoring over 24 hours, but shorter test durations produce similarly valid results, the analysis being either time-related or frequency-dependent.

The time-related method uses either heart rates measured at predefined times or the intervals between subsequent or chronologically unrelated RR-intervals for the analysis. Simple measurement results include the average duration of RR-intervals, or the mean heart rate taken at various times, or the difference between the shortest and the longest RR-interval. The most common measurement or reference value is the standard deviation of the total number of determined NN-intervals (SDNN). NN-intervals (nor-

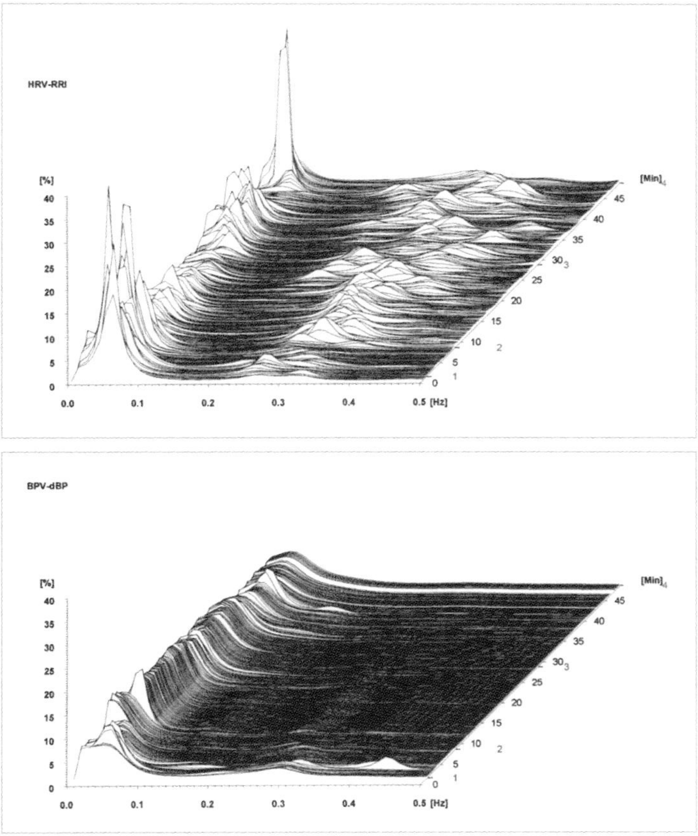

Figure 4 Three-dimensional diagram of the frequency-spectra of heart rate and blood pressure.

mal-to-normal) are defined as RR-intervals between QRS-complexes following a depolarization of the sinus node. The inclusion of further parameters can yield various additional values [307].

The results of spectral analysis of heart rate and blood pressure can be presented by means of three-dimensional diagrams (Fig. 4).

In order to adjust to changing demands in predefined periods of time, there are rhythmic and periodical fluctuations in heart rate and blood pressure. The frequency-related analysis, or spectral analysis, is able to detect slow fluctuations as well as rapid rhythmic changes. Signals of cardiovascular origin are repeated in every single heartbeat, without occurring at constant times. Morphology, amplitude and phase are variable end results of complex regulatory mechanisms. Under steady-state conditions the signals occur around an assessable mean value as an interpretable parameter. By means of the mathematic models of the Fourier transformation and of autoregressive methods, hidden rhythmic fluctuations can be detected in a seemingly chaotic heart rate course, yielding three impressive frequency spectra: high frequency changes of heart rate ranging around 0.25 Hz (HF-oscillations between 0.15 and 0.4 Hz), low frequency changes ranging around 0.1 Hz (LF-oscillations between 0.04 and 0.15 Hz) and very low fluctuations (VLF-oscillations between 0.003 and 0.04 Hz) ranging around 0.01 Hz.

The physiological basis of HF-oscillations is found in vagally mediated and respiration-dependent fluctuations of RR-intervals. LF-oscillations are created by the adjustment of RR-intervals to changes in blood pressure mediated by the baroreceptor reflex, whereas very slow rhythmic fluctuations of heart rate (VLF-oscillations) represent thermoregulatory adjustment processes and hormonal changes, namely via the renin-angiotensin-aldosterone system.

An intact autonomic regulatory function is reflected in the easy recognition of every single frequency range. Malfunctions of the autonomic circulatory regulation system result in altered spectra and the proportion of a frequency in the total spectrum, the so-called power, changes. The power spectral densities (PSD) of the LF- and HF-components are quantitative indicators of the autoregulatory function, their ratio (LF/HF ratio) represents the sympatho-vagal balance.

The normal values of heart rate variability and baroreflex sensitivity are limited because they are influenced by fluctuations related to time of the day, several candidate-related parameters and the implemented measuring method. The method of spectral analysis has proved to be the most stable parameter with the best reproducibility [186]. Nevertheless, tests should be performed, as far as possible, under similar conditions and at the same times of the day.

1.5.3 Evaluation of cardiovascular autonomic function

A number of maneuvers during non-invasive hemodynamic monitoring and tilt table testing provide insight into the reflex arcs of the autonomic nervous system. Diseases of the autonomic nervous system in combination with orthostatic intolerance are classified into acute and chronic, primary and secondary dysfunctions (Table 5).

While clinical symptoms rarely become manifest in the early stages of a disease, clinical tests enable the early detection of autonomic neuropathies. In patients with type II diabetes mellitus, subclinical neuropathy can be detected within one year of onset of the disease, and in patients with type I diabetes within two years. Orthostatic hypotension is often an indication of autonomic dysfunction that has progressed. 25–50% of diabetics with symptomatic autonomic dysfunction die within 5–10 years. The 5-year mortality in diabetics with autonomic dysfunction is three times higher than in diabetics without detectable abnormality of the autonomic nervous system [319,334].

As stated in the previous chapter, changes in heart rate or the RR-interval should be monitored carefully, with particular emphasis on responses to various stimulating agents. These include pharmacologic vasoconstrictive or vasodilative substances, orthostatic stress (lying, standing, squatting), respiratory tests including the Valsalva maneuver, coughing, thermal stress, or physical exercise

Table 5 Causes of autonomic dysfunctions with orthostatic intolerance

Primary autonomic dysfunctions	**Secondary autonomic dysfunctions**
• Acute pandysautonomia • Pure autonomic failure • Multiple system atrophy • Neurally mediated reflex syncope	*Central causes* • Brain tumors • Multiple sclerosis • Syringobulbia *Peripheral disorders* *Afferent* • Guillain-Barré syndrome • Posterior spinal sclerosis • Adie's syndrome *Efferent* • Diabetes mellitus • Deficit of neural insulin-like growth factors • Dopamine-beta-hydroxylases deficit *Afferent and efferent* • Hereditary dysautonomia *Spinal localization* • Myelitis • Syringomelia • Tumors *Other causes* • Renal insufficiency • Paraneoplastic syndromes • Collagenoses • Autoimmune diseases • HIV • Amyloidosis • Drug-induced

with subsequent metabolic changes to provoke a sympathicotonic response. A popular series of tests is known as the "Ewing Battery" [85], which will be described in the practical section of this book (Chapter 2.2.3).

The most frequently encountered tests include deep respiration, active orthostasis and the Valsalva maneuver. The various stages of these tests enable the selective recognition of the sympathetic and the parasympathetic components of the autonomic nervous system.

It is important that tests of the cardiovascular autonomic function utilize the continuous monitoring of blood pressure and heart rate.

1.5.3.1 Deep breathing

Respiratory arrhythmias are associated with a stimulation of cardioinhibitory centers in the medulla oblongata during the process of breathing. Inspiration increases the heart rate, while expiration decreases it. This mechanism is thought to be mediated by the Bainbridge reflex. During inspiration local muscle spindles in the right atria emit signals that cause inhibition of tone of the vagus nerve and excitation of the cardiac accelerator nerves leading to a subsequent rise in heart rate.

Testing consists of an individual performing controlled breathing with 6 deep breaths per minute. The shortest RR interval during inspiration (I) and the longest RR-interval during expiration (E) are analyzed to yield a resulting heart rate. A difference (E/I-difference) of >15 bpm is regarded as normal, values below 10 beats are considered abnormal, indicating a reduced adaptation. The E/I-ratio defines the quotient of E and I, and is highly age-related.

1.5.3.2 Active orthostasis

The change from a supine to a standing posture triggers complex reactions of the autonomic nervous system that consist of several phases.

The first phase is defined by a sudden increase in heart rate with a first peak after 3 s caused by an inhibition of vagal tone, followed by the second phase that has a less drastic increase and a peak after 12 s, which is followed by a baroreflex-mediated increase in heart rate. An over-reaction of compensatory mechanisms in the third phase can trigger transient bradycardia. Parasympathetic blocking after administration of atropine, as well as cardiovagal dysfunction of other origins, leads to the absence of the reactions of the first and third phase.

The 30:15 ratio has been validated as a quantifiable parameter for the intact function of the mentioned reflex arc. This ratio is the quotient of the shortest RR-interval at approximately the 15th beat after standing and the longest interval after approximately the 30th beat after standing. Normal values are highly age-related (see Chapter 2.2.3).

1.5.3.3 Valsalva maneuver

Similar to the regulatory mechanisms of active orthostasis, the adaptation processes of the autonomic nervous system during hemodynamic adjustments to increased intrathoracic pressure also consist of several phases.

In the first phase (phase I) the intrathoracic pressure rise causes compression of the aorta and a subsequent increase of blood pressure. This phase lasts only 1–4 s.

The early stage of the second phase (phase IIa) is defined by an impaired venous return, generating a fall in cardiac output and blood pressure, which then activates the baroreceptor reflex, leading to a rise in heart rate and in peripheral resistance due to sympathetically mediated vasoconstriction, and thus to subsequent recovery of blood pressure (phase IIb).

Upon cessation of expiration there is a mechanically induced fall in blood pressure (phase III), before the Valsalva maneuver ends (phase IV) with an abrupt drop of intrathoracic pressure, followed by an increase in cardiac output and blood pressure caused by restored venous return, and a subsequent compensatory decrease in heart rate.

In practice the test should be repeated several times in order to yield a clear-cut documentable result. The reference value for its analysis is the so-called Valsalva-ratio. It is the quotient of the longest RR-interval after the maneuver and of the shortest RR-interval during or immediately after the maneuver. Normal values are varied and dependant upon age.

1.5.3.4 Heart rate variability during orthostatic stress

The assessment of time-related or frequency-dependent parameters of heart rate variability during tilt table testing may point to autonomic control disturbances in patients with syncope [220].

The autonomic nervous system shows different reactions in healthy individuals and patients with syncope. Furlan [98] describes two different response patterns of the autonomic parameters LFnu, HFnu and LF/HF of heart rate variability in young patients with vasovagal syncopes:

The "sudden syncope" pattern is characterized by a progressive increase in sympathetic nerve activity (LFnu) during tilting, until the time of a sudden onset of bradycardia. Mosquedo-Garcia [226] and Moack [316] also observed an increase in sympathetic nerve activity, followed by a sudden drop immediately before the onset of syncope.

The "syncope with latency" pattern is characterized by a periodical inhibited sympathetic nerve activity (LFnu) accompanied by an increase in vagal nerve activity (HFnu) during passive orthostasis. In this pattern, Moack [216] also observed that during tilting a more distinctive and earlier decrease of LFnu in blood pressure fluctuation than in heart rate fluctuation occured.

In patients with vasovagal syncope Morillo [220] detected a slowed power rise in the LF-range and an increased power in the HF-range after moving to the upright position, corresponding to Furlan's second pattern. This might demonstrate a possible key role of the Bezold-Jarisch reflex in the onset of syncope [218]. The mechanism is a cardiovascular decompressor reflex involving a marked increase in vagal efferent discharge to the heart, elicited by stimulation of chemoreceptors, primarily in the left ventricle. This causes a slowing of the heart beat and dilatation of peripheral blood vessels with resulting lowering of the blood pressure. The concept was originated by Bezold in 1867, later revised by Jarisch in 1937.

The reduction of the sympatho-vagal balance (LF/HF) to <6 after 5 minutes of upright posture may represent a clear predictor for an imminent onset of a syncopal episode, which might render more time-intensive protocols useless.

1.5.3.5 Sustained handgrip test

Isometric contraction of the hand causes a rise in blood pressure and heart rate. This mechanism represents an efferent response of the sympathetic system. A rise in systolic blood pressure of >16 mmHg is regarded as normal, whereas increases <10 mmHg are considered abnormal.

1.5.4 Optimization of dual chamber cardiac pacemakers and cardiac resynchronization systems

The optimization of atrioventricular conduction time (AV-delay) leads to improvement in the hemodynamic situation in patients with dual chamber cardiac pacemakers [97,159] or devices for cardiac resynchronization [12].

There are various methods of AV-delay optimization: on the one hand Ritter's [192] echocardiographic method, on the other hand Koglek's formula of ECG (mostly lead V1), where the distance between the end of the P-wave and the R-peak (period of isovolumetric contraction) is calculated and "corrected" by an age-related value of 100–120 ms. The resulting difference is substracted from the existing AV-delay in order to achieve an "optimized AV-delay".

Another option is the method using transesophageal ECG that has been postulated by Ismer and Knorre [136].

In the setting of modern analysis-systems, impedance cardiography offers an additional, simple alternative. It has the potential to immediately control the success of reset of AV-delay by means of continuous graphic recording of cardiac output augmentation.

Chronic heart failure is associated with increased morbidity and mortality rates and is the most frequent cause for hospital admission in patients aged >65 years [182]. Cardiac resynchronization therapy by means of atrium-synchronized biventricular stimulation is an innovative procedure that has been established for therapeutic use in patients with mild or serious heart failure and intraventricular conduction system dysfunction. Early studies [103] have already demonstrated a long-term functional improvement. These encouraging findings have been validated by randomized controlled studies [4,45,182,330].

In those studies the efficacy of cardiac resynchronization with advanced echocardiographic and technological programming equipment has been refined and controlled. Considering the potential extent of this therapeutic procedures application, the simple optimization of hemodynamic features might be of substantial benefit. Here modern devices bringing together non-invasive blood pressure monitoring with impedance cardiography represent appropriate solutions. Such programs enable the continuous display of left ventricular function parameters (stroke volume, cardiac index, index of contractility, maximal rise in pressure), and thus the "on-line" and beat-to-beat control of the efficacy of re-programming a cardiac resynchronization system.

1.5.5 Sudden cardiac death and risk stratification

Martin [208] developed a method of risk stratification in patients with syncope, the primary outcome being the development of serious cardiac arrhythmias and/or sudden cardiac death. The identified 4 risk factors were age >45 years, history of serious cardiac arrhythmias or heart failure and abnormal resting-ECG. Development of the primary outcome occurred in only 4–7% of cases which did not have any of the risk factors, whilst it was 58–80% of cases in patients with three or more factors. The critical importance of identifying patients at risk of malignant arrhythmias and sudden cardiac death lies in the fact that a significant number of the underlying diseases are now treatable.

In those with a history of acute myocardial infarction, left ventricular dysfunction and ventricular arrhythmias are thought to almost double the mortality risk [196,321]. Experiments carried out in dogs have yielded the first indications of the influence of the autonomic nervous system on sudden cardiac death [27,284,287].

The key role of autonomic mechanisms comes from experimentally induced myocardial infarction which provoked ventricular fibrillation primarily in those dogs with reduced vagal reflexes and increased sympathetic activity. An observed increase in in-hospital mortality in patients after acute myocardial infarction who had reduced physiologic sinus arrhythmia has given rise to a number of connected studies [25,160,248].

Studies in human patients have demonstrated the role of impaired baroreflex sensitivity [87,173] as well as of reduced heart rate variability [6,25,157,248] in predicting cardiac mortality after acute myocardial infarction.

Reduced vagal activity, derived from baroreflex sensitivity and heart rate variability with subsequent sympathetic dominance, is a serious risk factor [27,179,287]. The arrhythmogenic potential of sympathetic hyperactivity is well-known [286]. In this respect, vagal stimulation may have an antagonistic effect. Baroreflex sensitivity is also a quantifiable variable of the ability to augment parasympathetic tone [171].

Findings of smaller studies [87,173] demonstrating an association between impaired baroreflex sensitivity and mortality risk after acute myocardial infarction, have led to a multi-center prospective study in 1,284 patients of myocardial infarction within 28 days. The ATRAMI study [168] demonstrated that during a follow-up of 21 months reduced heart rate variability (SDNN <70 ms) and reduced baroreflex sensitivity (<3.0 ms/mmHg) had a significant influence on an increased risk of sudden cardiac death. If both parameters ranged below the mentioned values, the examined patients displayed a 2-year mortality of 17%, in contrast to a respective mortality rate of only 2% if both parameters were normal (SDNN >105 ms, BRS >6.1 ms/mmHg). Impaired baroreflex sensitivity and heart rate variability were identified as major risk factors, independent of the seriousness of impaired left ventricular function or of the presence of ventricular arrhythmias.

In addition to the time-related parameter SDNN, frequency-related parameters of heart rate variability can also be used for cardiac risk stratification [201]. In this context the reduction of low frequency units <0.04 Hz are of crucial importance. Other studies have demonstrated the importance of VLF values and of even lower frequency spectra (ULF – ultra low frequency) [25]. In patients with heart failure, VLF-power and NYHA-classification, presence of diabetes mellitus and the serum concentration of brain natriuretic peptide can be considered as independent predictors of an increased risk of cardiac death [128].

In addition to the parameters of impaired left ventricular function or of serious arrhythmias, heart rate variability (SDNN) and baroreflex sensitivity can be used to further evaluate patients with normal ranges of the mentioned values, in order to obtain an individualized optimization of risk stratification.

During the acute phase of myocardial infarction there is a significant association between reduced SDNN, the degree of left ventricular dysfunction and the peak serum level of creatine kinase [53]. Various hypotheses have attempted to explain this phenomenon: One possible association may be related to the changed ventricular geometry after myocardial infarction with altered cardiac tension sensors and subsequently increased cardiac sympathetic tone [47,203]. A further hypothesis is based on the assumption of impaired sinus node reactivity due to influences of the autonomous nervous system [202,287]. In addition, changed intracardiac sympatho-vagal reflexes are thought to be a possible cause [285].

La Rovere [172] demonstrated that in patients with heart failure even a short-term reduction of HRV, namely a reduction of LF-values to <11–13 ms^2 can be considered an independent marker of sudden cardiac death. In this study time-related and frequency-related parameters of heart rate variability were recorded in the supine position by means of ECG over 8 minutes with a predetermined respiration rate of 12–15/min. Calculation was based on autoregressive mathematical methods and the determination of SDNN (time-related) and LF/HF values (frequency-related).

The results of this study confirmed a 3-year-mortality rate of sudden cardiac death of 23% in the group with low LF-power, compared to a rate by 7% among patients with preserved LF-values. In summary, the combination of preserved LF-values with an absence of serious cardiac arrhythmias resulted in a patient subgroup with a 3-year-mortality rate ranging as low as 3%. Hypotheses concerning reduced LF-power include potentially reduced sinus node reactivity, absent oscillation ability during prolonged sympathetic hyperactivity [225], failure of central regulatory mechanisms [238,316] as well as the influence of reduced baroreflex sensitivity [293]. The latter is known to be involved in LF-range undulations.

Heart rate variability is known to be reduced not only in patients with acute myocardial infarction but also in the clinical setting of various other cardiac and non-cardiac clinical conditions [307]: heart transplantation, congenital heart failure, chronic mitral regurgitation, mitral valve prolapse syndrome, supraventricular or ventricular tachycardia, anti-arrhythmic therapy or diabetic neuropathy. In addition, physical exercise can lead to a rise in SDNN [134]. Opinions regarding the beneficial effects of drugs like betablockers or scopolamine or of thrombolysis in the case of acute myocardial infarctions are divided [5,169,281,332]. Considering the immediate physiological changes after an acute myocardial infarction it is not recommended that a patient's heart rate variability is measured until a week after the infarction [307].

In view of a sufficient number of randomized studies and meta-analyses, the guidelines of the European Society of Cardiology include a Class I recommendation for the assessment of baroreflex sensitivity and heart rate variability as independent prognostic markers of sudden cardiac death.

There is hope that in the future there will be the development of individualized risk stratifications based on the inclusion of parameters of autonomic (time-related analysis of heart rate variability (SDNN), LF-power during a frequency-dependent spectral analysis of heart rate variability, baroreflex sensitivity) and non-autonomic cardiovascular functions (left ventricular ejection fraction, plasma-pro-NT-BNP level, plasma-noradrenaline level, etc.).

1.5.6 Therapeutic follow-up

1.5.6.1 Neurally mediated reflex syncope – therapeutic follow-up

Tilt table and domestic tilt training are the therapeutic measures that are recommended [78,83].

Considering the acceptable reproducibility of tilt table testing it is suitable for therapeutic control of neurally mediated reflex syncope. This may result in therapeutic modifications, or, in the case of a negative response, differential-diagnostic considerations.

In spite of positive findings [126], the unrestricted use of tilt table testing for therapeutic follow-up should be considered cautiously because of the methodological problems that have been described above.

1.5.6.2 Therapeutic optimization after acute myocardial infarction

There are now a wide range of standard therapeutic drugs for patients who present with acute myocardial infarction. In high-risk patients, an extended profile of therapeutic measures might be recommended.

The evaluation of baroreflex sensitivity and heart rate variability may enable first the identification of high-risk patients, and second, the therapeutic assessment of standard or extended therapeutic measures.

The latter comprise not only of the use of beta-blockers, but also of other anti-arrhythmic drugs and of implantable uni- or biventricular defibrillators.

An interesting approach is the administration of concentrated omega-3-fatty acids. A small study on post-infarction patients showed enhanced heart rate variability after 12 weeks of omega-3-fatty acid intake [56]. A subsequent study demonstrated a positive correlation between levels of omega-3-fatty acids in the membrane of granulocytes and enhanced heart rate variability [57]. The GISSI-P-study [81] confirmed the clearest evidence so far of the beneficial effect of omega-3-fatty acids. 11,324 post-infarction patients were administered either vitamin E and/or omega-3-fatty acids (460 mg Eicosapentaen acid and 380 mg Docosahexaen acid) or placebo in addition to usual therapeutic measures. After 3.5 years the patient group that had been treated with omega-3-fatty acids showed a 30% diminution of cardiovascular mortality and a sudden cardiac death rate reduction of 45%. The physical correlation of these findings may lie in an anti-arrhythmic and anti-fibrillation effect accompanied by the inhibition of sodium and calcium ion-influx, with subsequent hyperpolarization of the resting-membrane-potential with an electric stabilization of myocardial cells. Further increases in heart rate variability may be achieved by physical exercise [28,134,244].

The increased sympathetic activity accompanied by a reduced influence of parasympathetic activity is a characteristic marker of high-risk patients after myocardial infarction. Apart from the established use of beta-blockers selective cardiac muscarine-receptor-antagonists might also play a significant future role.

The findings of heart rate variability and baroreflex sensitivity evaluation may prove useful for therapeutic follow-up, but might also become a key factor in the identification of patients for more aggressive anti-arrhythmic therapeutic procedures.

1.5.7 Non-invasive evaluation of parameters of cardiovascular function in diagnosis and monitoring

The high degree of correlation between invasive blood pressure and hemodynamic features measured by cannulation, and non-invasive blood pressure monitoring [170] by means of finger-plethysmography and impedance cardiography [20,21,317] advocates their extended use in all areas where there is a need for continuous and complete monitoring.

The complications of invasive methods like infections and tissue injuries are well known. The costs of material and patient care are further factors arguing in favor of non-invasive methods.

Other potential uses of this novel technology would include intensive care units and intra- and perioperative monitoring.

1.6 Outlook – general comments

Combined methods to evaluate hemodynamic features and individual cardiovascular autonomic values are a simple, non-invasive, bedside assessment technique that obtains valuable data for patient monitoring.

Apart from possible uses for patient surveillance (intensive care, surgery), impedance cardiography and non-invasive blood pressure monitoring by means of finger-plethysmography may also be of use in telemedical settings. At present, several signals can be transferred, but there is no device currently available that is able to transmit a variety of hemodynamic parameters and ECG-data at the same time. Wave charts in the form of external loop recorders or implantable devices are able to transmit ECGs, but the second crucial parameter, blood pressure, is not transmitted. The current ability to digitize simple, continuous and non-invasive blood pressure evaluation by finger cuff measuring, is the basis for its future transmittance.

Fascinating new fields of application include telemedical disciplines, namely tele-cardiology. Possible uses including combination of mobile phone technologies, GPRS (General Packet Radio Service), GPS (Global Positioning System) and digitized bio-signals which are transmitted by implanted or external devices are at the forefront of emerging research [236].

In 1997, Aaronson [1] developed a method to assess the urgency of the need for heart transplantation. In this respect parameters obtained by simple and non-invasive techniques were equally valid, compared with those obtained by traditional methods. In view of the availability and cost-effectiveness this also argues in favor of non-invasive methods. While single values are of limited use [1,307], a variable combination of independent parameters may yield a high degree of predictive value. Studies have demonstrated that among 80 evaluated clinical features a combination of 7 parameters proved to be the most appropriate to predict the mortality risk of cardiac transplantation candidates: presence of ischemic cardiomyopathy, resting heart-rate, left ventricular ejection fraction, QRS duration >0.12 s, mean arterial blood pressure, maximal oxygen-intake and serum sodium level.

A similarly differentiated score-system for risk stratification of post-infarction patients does not exist so far. Some groups are associated with a clear-cut increased mortality risk [10,50,60,61,59, 102,106,150,155,181,195,273,302,315]. But so far, there exists no comprehensive risk stratification that includes parameters of the non-autonomic and autonomic functions. Such stratification might determine highly individualized therapeutic recommendations, which might be included in future guidelines.

When considering overall mortality, the predictive value of impaired heart rate variability is equal to that of reduced left ventricular ejection fraction, but it is of superior value in predicting sudden cardiac death related to ventricular arrhythmia [248]. These findings are of significant importance for the value of parameters of cardiovascular control, namely heart rate variability and baroreflex sensitivity.

There are currently a wide range of available treatment options. Changes of life-style, pharmacological treatment, as well as implantable resynchronization systems and defibrillators are efficient therapeutic tools. However, using non-invasive tests of cardiovascular autonomic functions in the identification of patients for whom further therapeutic measures are appropriate is a relatively young field.

Based on studies in the early 1980s indicating that fetal stress might be reflected in changed RR-intervals [132], advanced methods of power spectral analysis might enable insights into early infantile control of cardiovascular autonomic functions. Assessment of heart rate variability and baroreflex sensitivity could play a key role in risk stratifications of sudden infant death.

It is a well known fact that the administration of atropine leads to a reduction of heart rate variability, while the transdermal administration of scopolamine has the opposite effect, which indicates the potential possibility of modulating autonomic parameters by means of pharmacological intervention. But in spite of promising experimental findings it has not been possible to demonstrate the efficacy of scopolamine to avoid ventricular fibrillation in dogs after acute myocardial infarction. Beta-blockers have rarely been studied in this situation, but in an experimental study no benefit could be demonstrated [5]. Currently available non-invasive methods of assessing heart rate variability, determining sympathetic and parasympathetic functions, analyzing baroreflex sensitivity, as well as assessing cardiovascular hemodynamics have considerably simplified the trial process for new pharmacological therapies. New therapeutic strategies incorporating a modification of the autonomic nervous system to enhance parasympathetic function and to impede sympathetic function are being scientifically discussed.

The symptom complex of syncope is a clear example of uneconomical diagnostic processes. Injuries due to falling are a serious problem for older patients. There are estimations about a yearly incidence of femoral neck fractures ranging around 1.5 million worldwide [124], with an estimated mortality rate of about 25%. This number is expected to rise to 2.5 million accidents in 2025. For this type of accident alone the yearly medical costs are 7.2 billion USD, with an estimated rise to 16 billions per year by 2040.

Advanced electronic and paper-based expert systems (clinical pathways) are indispensable future measures to avoid obsolete diagnostic procedures and to promote algorithm-controlled decisions.

1.7 Summary

The combined use of non-invasive methods of continuous beat-to-beat blood pressure monitoring, impedance cardiography and tilt table testing allow the assessment of a comprehensive profile of individual hemodynamic and autonomic cardiovascular parameters.

In addition to its traditional field of application, namely management of syncope, there are is a wide range of current or future innovative applications in cardiology and related disciplines, which will allow clinical medicince to cope with the growing challenges of medical quality and economic use of limited resources.

2 Practical application and protocols

Dependent upon the hard- and software systems that are chosen, a variety of results can be obtained[1].

Considering the high number of potential scientific applications, the following chapter is restricted to the essential fields of clinical relevance. These comprise: syncope diagnosis, assessment of baroreflex sensitivity, heart rate variability and hemodynamic parameters, and – as an extension of routine patient work-ups – functional testing of the autonomic nervous system. The utilization of non-invasive monitoring in order to optimize cardiac pacemaker settings will also be briefly reviewed.

2.1 Recommendations for tilt table test procedures

2.1.1 Preparation

The following should be observed when preparing a patient for a tilt table test (see Chapter 1.2.7.2.3).

1. *Patients should be well informed and should fast for at least 2 hours before the test, preferably overnight.*

Patient information should refer to individual indications, the date set for the test, as well as protocol details. The fact that a synco-

[1] The practical applications described in this chapter are based on the utilization of the Task Force® Monitor by the Austrian company CNSystems Medizintechnik GmbH (www.cnsystems.at). The graphics and data displayed herein are the sole results of using the Task Force® Monitor.

pal episode could occur and that the present staff will ensure its prompt interruption by returning the patient to the supine position should be explained to the patient in detail. In addition, typical side-effects associated with the possible use of provocative agents should be emphasized. The use of glyceryl trinitrate, for instance, entails typical side-effects like headache, vertigo, light-headedness, nausea and vomiting. In the case of a planned isoprotenerol challenge the patient should be specifically informed about the possibility of cardiac arrhythmias.

Repeated tests should preferably be performed at the same time of the day in order to ensure consistency of circadian influences. Morning appointments are recommended thus allowing the patient to fast overnight. If the tests are performed at other times, the patient should fast for at least two hours prior to tilt table testing [33].

2. *The room should be quiet and with a constant comfortable temperature.*

In order to prevent external disturbing influences, a constantly maintained temperature and a quiet environment are recommended to ensure comparable test conditions. The baseline autonomous tone is of critical importance in cardiovascular autonomic function testing.

3. *Continuous beat-to-beat monitoring of blood pressure and heart rate, as well as constant ECG monitoring.*

Non-invasive blood pressure measurement by means of the vascular unloading technique enables continuous beat-to-beat monitoring. Intermittent blood pressure monitoring using upper arm cuffs is not recommended, particularly given the difficulties in differentiating and classifying a possible syncopal spell and the need to analyze cardiovascular autonomic parameters.

4. *Immediately available physician*

The low incidence of serious complications does not warrant attendance of a physician. He/she should, however, be available within the immediate vicinity of the test in case of symptom development or complications.

5. *Immediately available resuscitation team and equipment.*
Medical staff (a nurse or a medical technician) should be in attendance during the entire test procedure to monitor the patient, control vital functions, to perform various tests or to prevent technical errors like a dislocated measurement device. In case of serious complication, a physician should be immediately available. Resuscitation equipment includes the standard emergency equipment enabling defibrillation, ventilatory support, oxygen supply and pharmacological therapy.

6. *Supine position for a minimum of 5 minutes before tilting, and for at least 20 minutes if vascular cannulation is employed.*
This equilibration period is recommended [33] in order to minimize disturbing influences caused by preparation procedures after transport and patient positioning, or after connecting the patient to the measurement devices. The influence of intravenous cannulation on the cardiovascular autonomic tone necessitates a considerably longer supine phase.

7. *Tilt table of the foot-board support type, angles should be able to be set quickly as well as slowly.*
A foot-board prevents the patient from slipping down, and, like a restraining strap placed across the abdomen, it is an indispensable and common part of modern tilt tables. For diagnostic purposes, angles should be able to be set slowly and smoothly, however, after a documented positive test response or in case of complications, it should be possible to reset the tilt table quickly to the supine position.

2.1.2 Proposed protocol

There is a wide variety of tilt table testing protocols in existence, differing in time duration of the various phases, tilt angles, use of provocative agents and the analysis of the performed tests. Tests for scientific purposes or tests for the evaluation of the cardiovascular autonomic function may warrant different protocols.

The test procedure may be shortened by refraining from evaluating hemodynamic baseline values and baroreflex sensitivity and by laying an emphasis on unmasking the underlying cause of syncope. The protocol mentioned below describes an individualized evaluation process resulting from the combination of various existing protocols that takes into consideration individual test sensitivity and specificity and the numerous possibilities offered by the combination of tilt table testing, impedance cardiography and continuous non-invasive blood pressure monitoring.

Protocol

The patient assumes the position on the tilt table, and the measurement devices are applied. Subsequently a rest/equilibration period of at least 10 minutes – or of at least 20 minutes if vascular cannulation is employed – should be observed to ensure that the autonomic tone is not influenced or disturbed by transport and preparation procedures. However, this equilibration period may be shortened, if attention is paid to a clear HF-waveband displayed in the graphic view of heart rate analysis, which can be considered as a sign of the patient having "settled in". Only then can the measuring phase begin.

Next, a measuring period of 10 minutes with the patient lying supine is recommended to obtain baseline hemodynamic parameters by means of impedance cardiography, as well as the parameters of the cardiovascular autonomic state (i.e., baroreflex sensitivity). The advocated duration of 10 minutes allows an easy conversion of the obtained values into per-minute-values.

After that the patient is tilted in a slow and steady motion to an upright position at an angle of 60°. If no symptoms occur within 20 minutes the patient is challenged with a dose of glyceryl trinitate spray (400 µg). If after this drug challenge no positive response occurs the patient is to stay upright for another 20 minutes. When there is a positive response to tilting it is of integral importance to in the first instance ask the patient whether the present symptoms correspond to the definition of a true syncopal attack, and secondly, to wait for a clear and indisputable hemodynamic response (i.e., it would be best to wait for a true syncopal attack). Premature interruption often leads to ambiguous results which might subsequently cast doubts on a potential diagnosis. As soon as unmistakable symptoms occur, the tilt table is set quickly to the supine position. Depending on the patient's regaining consciousness and his/her circulatory condition, the test may be terminated after 5 minutes, but if necessary, the patient may require a longer recovery phase.

Table 6 Possible chronological course of a tilt table test

Action	Duration/min
Application of measurement devices	
Equilibration phase in supine position	10
Measurement phase in supine position	10
Tilting, upright posture until drug challenge*	20
Administration of 400 µg glyceryl trinitate	
Upright posture after drug challenge*	20
Resetting to supine position, recovery	5

* if no symptoms have been observed

2.2 Evaluation

2.2.1 Physiological reaction in response to orthostatic stress

A physiological reaction to orthostatic stress comprises the following hemodynamic changes:

- Increase in heart rate (HR) by 10–20 bpm

The heart rate is determined by means of ECG recordings.

- Fall in systolic blood pressure (BP) by 0–10 mmHg

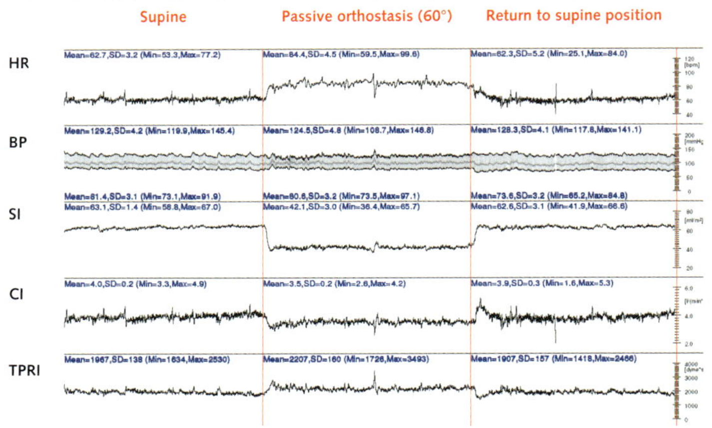

Figure 5 Physiological behavior of heart rate (HR), blood pressure (BP), stroke index (SI), cardiac index (CI) and total peripheral resistance index (TPRI) when lying supine and in upright position.

- Increase in diastolic blood pressure by 5–10 mmHg

Blood pressure is recorded non-invasively and continuously, by means of finger cuff recording using the "vascular unloading" technique (see Chapter 1.3).

- Decrease in stroke volume (and a drop in the body surface area related stroke index [SI9) of up to 35%

Stroke volume and the index related to body surface area are obtained from impedance cardiography signals and then calculated by means of mathematical modulation.

Cardiac output (CO) (L/min) and cardiac index (L/min/m^2) are subsequently derived parameters on a 1-minute-basis.

- Decrease in cardiac index (CI) of up to 20%

Cardiac index is a value calculated by means of impedance cardiography using the parameters of stroke volume, heart rate (HR) and body surface area (SV×HR/m^2). In spite of a fall in stroke volume the cardiac index is not reduced to the same extent as the stroke index, a phenomenon due to heart rate increase.

- Increase in total peripheral resistance (index) (TPRI) of up to 25%

Total peripheral resistance is a value derived from mean arterial blood pressure (MABP) (obtained via "vascular unloading" technique), central venous pressure (CVP, set for 3 mmHg) and cardiac output (CO), using the following formula: $[(MABP - CVP) : CO] \times 80$.

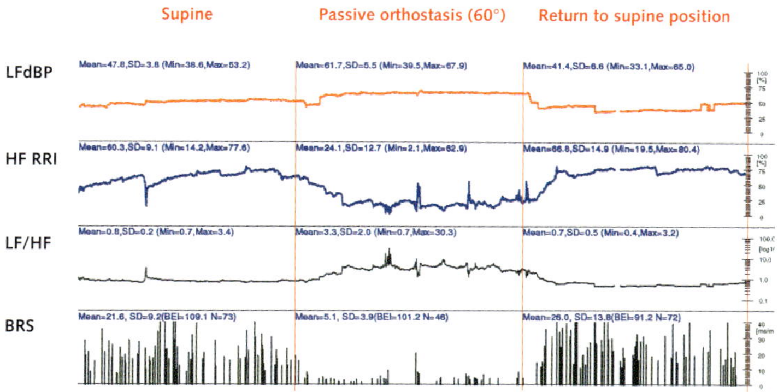

Figure 6 Physiological behavior of frequency components of sympathetic activity which regulate blood pressure (LF dBP), of vagal activity in the heart rate spectrum (HF_RRI), of the sympatho-vagal balance (LF/HF) and of baroreflex sensitivity in both supine and upright positions.

During orthostasis the parameters of the cardiovascular autonomic function and of the hemodynamic system are subject to multiple changes.

For normal values of the standard parameters of LF_RRI, LFnu_RRI, HF_RRI, HFnu_RRI and of power spectral density (PSD_RRI) as a benchmark parameter of spectral distribution (see Appendix 4.3). The suffix "nu" stands for "normalized units" and represents the relative distribution of a section of the frequency spectrum in relation to the total measured spectrum minus the VLF-components (thus the calculation operation for LFnu_RRI, for instance, is: LF_RRI/(Total Power – VLF_RRI) × 100).

- Increase in sympathetic activity regulating blood pressure (and heart rate [not applied here]) (LF dBP)

Orthostatic stress entails a prevalence of sympathicotonic counterregulation in order to maintain a sufficient mean systemic arterial blood pressure, leading to tachycardia and peripheral vasoconstriction.

The share of sympathicotonic activities to regulate blood pressure is assessed by detecting low frequency undulations within the spectrum of the blood pressure curve by means of autoregressive parameters. The displayed value represents the percentage of sympathicotonic regulatory activities in relation to the totality of blood pressure regulating activities.

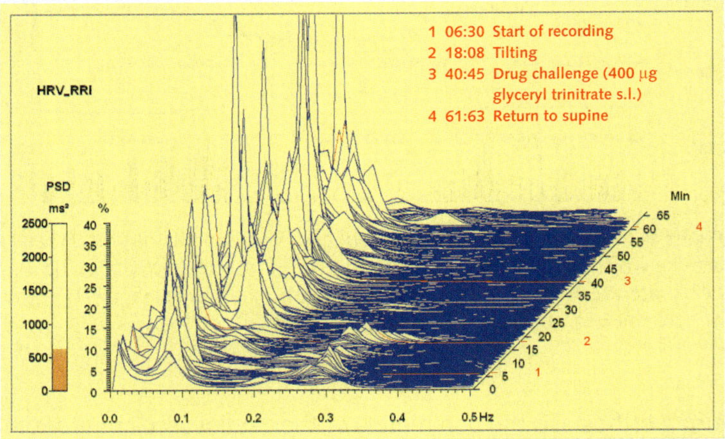

Figure 7 Diagram of physiological behavior of cardiovascular autonomous heart rate control (HRV_RRI). During phase 1 (rest) both frequency components are clearly detectable: the lower amplitudes of the vagal function (HF, ranging around 0.15–0.4 Hz) and the greater amplitudes of the sympathetic function (LF, ranging around 0.04–0.15 Hz). During phase 2 (tilting) and 3 (upright posture after administration of 400 µg GTN sublingually for drug challenge) the vagal component of the HF-regulation spectrum disappears, while the occurring orthostatic stress is marked by a dominance of the sympathetic component. Only after resetting the tilt table to the supine position (phase 4) does the vagal frequency range reappear.

• Decrease in vagal activity regulating the heart rate (HF_RRI)
Analogous to the prevalence of sympathetic activity during orthostatic stress, a baroreceptor reflex mediated withdrawal of vagal influence is generated within the heart rate spectrum.

The displayed value represents the percentage of vagal regulatory activities in relation to the totality of heart rate regulating activities.

Figure 7 shows a three-dimensional diagram of physiological behavior with maintained vagal activity during rest and withdrawal of vagal tone and prevalence of sympathetic influence during orthostasis.

• Rise in sympatho-vagal balance (LF/HF)
This value results from the spectral power in the LF- and HF-ranges of blood pressure (BP) and heart rate (reciprocally: RR-interval [RRI]) recorded with the patient lying supine. During orthostasis these quotients are subject to change. By choosing blood pressure spectra or heart rate spectra it is possible to calculate various quotients, e.g.:

a) LF_RRI/HF_RRI (LF/HF)
Sympatho-vagal balance within the heart rate spectrum

Normal value (in supine position): < 2

b) LF_BP/HF_RRI
Sympatho-vagal balance between the low frequency component of the blood pressure spectrum and the high frequency component of the heart rate spectrum

Normal value (in supine position): <2

Due to the changes of the various frequency components mentioned above, their respective quotient (LF/HF) changes likewise by increasing during orthostasis. The respective ordinate has a logarithmic scale. During rest a quotient <2 is regarded as normal, during orthostasis an increase by double the amount is to be expected.

• Decrease in baroreflex sensitivity during orthostasis (BRS)
During the increased sympathetic activity accompanied by a rise in heart rate, a decrease in baroreflex sensitivity can be observed.

Baroreflex sensitivity is assessed by means of the spontaneous sequence method [22,251] using ECG heart rate recordings and continuous beat-to-beat finger blood pressure measurement, as described in Chapter 1.3.

Detected events (up- and down-events) are displayed as bars, whose heights reflect the slope, i.e., the amplitudes of the reflex responses in ms/mmHg.

The rest values displayed in Figure 6 (mean (slope) = 21.6 ms/mmHg, N (number of detected events) = 73 (within 10 minutes), can be regarded as normal, or even as exceeding the standard values for the age category around 18 years.

For normal values regarding baroreflex sensitivity, see Appendix 4.3.

The obtained values may vary according to sex, body mass index, heart rate, blood pressure, smoking, alcohol consumption, physical activity, underlying diseases, as well as the chosen test protocol, plus they are strictly age-related [148].

Considering the high number of influences on heart rate variability and the numerous different measurement methods in use, it is not possible to fix absolute normal values for the parameters of autonomic control (LF-dBP, HF-RRI, LF-RRI). In this respect the sympatho-vagal balance is a more valid marker.

The normal values displayed in the appendix were obtained in studies with smaller patient populations with spectral analysis being performed during 5 minutes in the supine position, and represent approximate values [307].

Comparative analyses of data obtained by means of impedance cardiography, non-invasive blood pressure monitoring, and heart rate enable the assessment of further hemodynamic parameters. For this purpose phase 2 of tilt table testing (supine phase, data measurement during 10 minutes) can provide baseline values. However, parameters may also be obtained without using tilt table tests, other possibilities are, e.g., monitoring in the setting of a medical intensive care unit or telemetric monitoring.

Other hemodynamic parameters are:

- Acceleration index (1/100 s^2)

The acceleration index is a parameter derived from impedance cardiography and represents the maximum acceleration of blood flow during systole.

- Index of contractility (1/1000 s)

The index of contractility is a parameter derived from impedance cardiography and represents the maximum blood flow during systole. It can be detected in the ICG-waveform diagram as the upward curve (P-wave) following the opening of the aortic valve.

- Maximum rise in pressure [dP/dt_{max}] (mmHg/s)

The maximum rise in pressure is a parameter derived from non-invasive continuous finger blood pressure monitoring and represents the steepest rise of the pressure measured in the pulse wave.

- Pulse pressure (mmHg)

Pulse pressure is defined as the difference between systolic and diastolic arterial blood pressure. Normal values range around 30–40 mmHg.

Numerous epidemiological studies have demonstrated the independent and significant role of pulse pressure as a risk factor for cardiovascular morbidity and mortality in patients >50 (60) years. In this respect pulse pressure values >60–65 mmHg accompanied by normal or only slightly elevated mean pressure represent a considerable risk for coronary morbidity and mortality, and when accompanied by significantly elevated mean or diastolic blood pressure they represent a serious risk for cerebrovascular morbidity and mortality. An increase in pulse pressure is caused by decreased compliance of bigger vessels, but also by a premature and intensified pulse wave reflection, which, on the other hand, is associated with stiff vessels, arteriosclerotic plaque and remodeling in the peripheral vessels.

For normal values, see Appendix 4.3.

2.2.2 Pathophysiological patterns

2.2.2.1 Positive test result: syncope

When interpreting the findings of a tilt table test, the physician has various directions in which to proceed. In the setting of syncope diagnosis, without doubt the most important question is whether a syncopal event has occurred during the work-up. The clinical presentation of the symptoms must correspond to the definition of the symptom complex (see Chapter 1.2.1). It is of crucial importance to find out whether the witnessed clinical manifestation truly corresponds to the diagnostically relevant symptoms, or if it is an accidentally obtained clinical presentation because in this case the established diagnosis may not be the clinically relevant one.

In addition, all symptoms reported by the patient should be noted carefully, and special attention should be devoted to prodromal presyncopal symptoms which – in the absence of classical syncope – are characteristic of postural orthostatic tachycardia syndrome.

2.2.2.1.1 Classification of syncope

If syncope occurs it may be classified by means of blood pressure and heart rate behavior (Tables 7, 8). One classification is the traditional one proposed by the VASIS group [306], an alternative is a classification according to blood pressure and heart rate behavior during the presyncopal phase [36]. However, to date there is no validated subgroup-specific and differentiated treatment strategy based on these classifications.

Graphic illustrations displaying long-term trends in blood pressure and heart rate allow an easy classification into one of the mentioned groups. If the resolution of a printout is not high enough, it is possible to reload and analyze a "short-trend" recording, which is particularly important for the analysis of minimal heart rate and asystole duration.

Table 7 VASIS classification [306]

Type I: mixed	Heart rate falls at time of syncope, but not to <40 bpm, or heart rate falls to <40 bpm but for <10 s with or without asystole for <3 s. Blood pressure falls before heart rate falls.
Type II a: Cardioinhibition without asystole	Heart rate falls to <40 bpm for >10 s without asystole for >3 s. Blood pressure falls before heart rate falls.
Type II b: Cardioinhibition with asystole	Asystole occurs for >3 s. Blood pressure falls before or concurrently with heart rate.
Type III: Vasodepressor	Heart rate does not fall by >10% from its baseline value at the time of syncope
Exception 1	Chronotropic incompetence: no heart rate rise of ≥ 10% from its baseline value during tilting
Exception 2	Excessive heart rate rise to >130 bpm immediately after tilting and during the entire duration of upright posture before syncope

Table 8 Classification according to Brignole [36] (presyncopal phase)

Type	Heart rate	Blood pressure
Classic vasovagal syncope pattern	Rapid increase, then constantly high level (physiologic during presyncopal phase)	Discrete systolic fall, constant diastole
Dysautonomic vasovagal syncope pattern	Initially little to no increase (no or little compensation)	Always fluctuating, never constantly compensated
Orthostatic intolerance pattern	Constant increase, no fall (no true syncope, but prolonged presyncope)	Constantly falling, always fluctuating

2.2.2.1.2 Examples

The following real-life examples represent classic patterns of tilt table test procedures. The typical waveform display justifies the diagnosis of syncope only when associated with the occurrence of symptoms typical of syncope (VASIS I–III) or prolonged presyncope (POTS).

a) Mixed type of syncope (VASIS I)

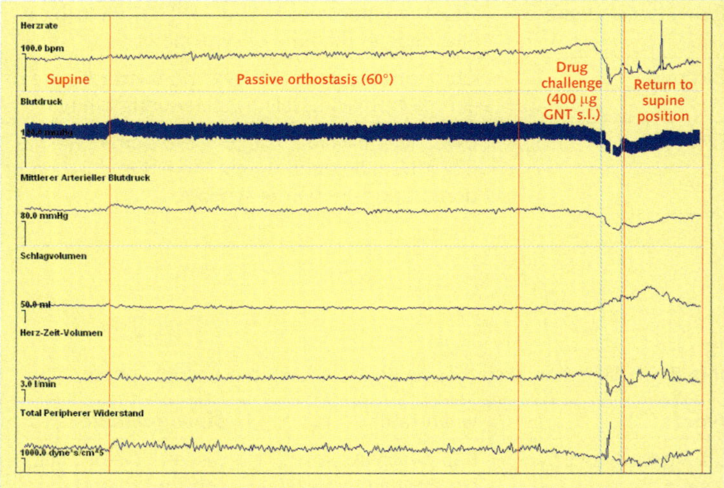

Figure 8 Progress of orthostatic response: Blood pressure fall occurs before heart rate decline, the latter remaining slightly above 40 bpm.

b) Cardioinhibitory syncope without asystole (VASIS IIa)

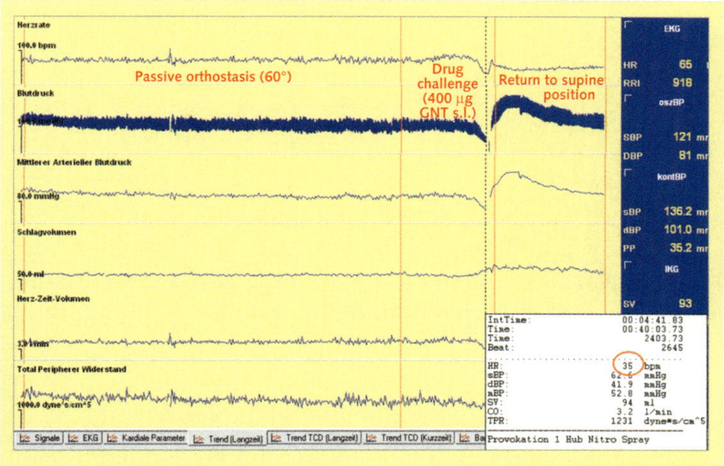

Figure 9 Progress of orthostatic response: Blood pressure fall occurs before heart rate fall, which declines below 40 bpm, but not below a minimum of 35 bpm (marker), and without asystole of >3 s.

c) Cardioinhibitory syncope with asystole (VASIS IIb)

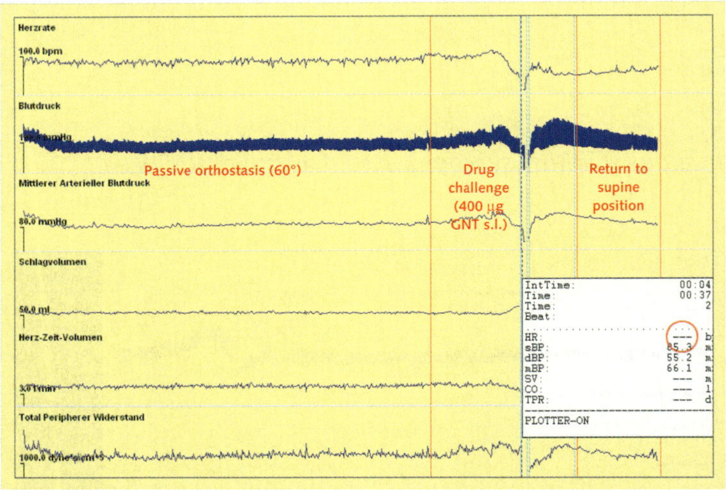

Figure 10 Progress of orthostatic response: Blood pressure fall and heart rate decline below 40 bpm, with asystole of >3 s.

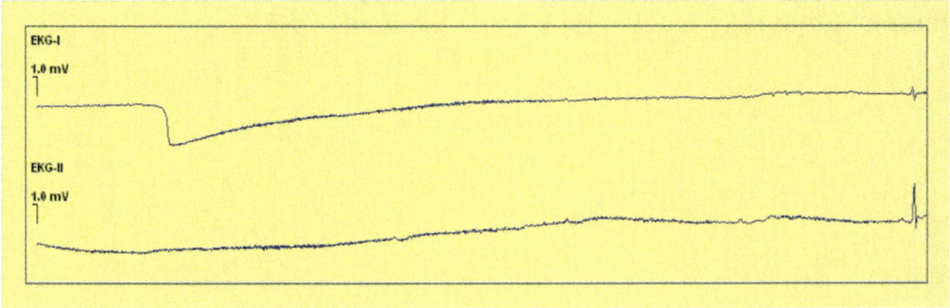

Figure 11 The exact analysis of the subtypes VASIS IIa or b necessitates a high-resolution ECG including minimal heart rate display. The duration of the displayed asystole was 26 s.

d) *Vasodepressor syncope (VASIS III)*

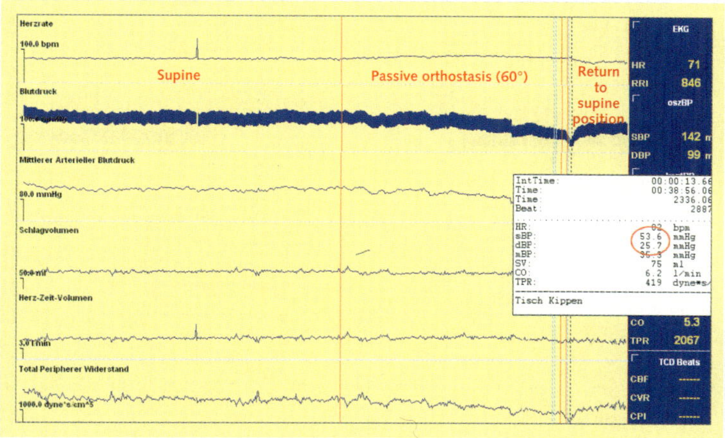

Figure 12 Progress of orthostatic response: isolated blood pressure fall to 54/26 mmHg (marker) without decline in heart rate (stable at 82 bpm). In this case no drug challenge was necessary. Syncope occurred after 12 minutes of upright posture, with prodromal symptoms occurring after 10 minutes.

2.2.2.2 Positive test result: POTS

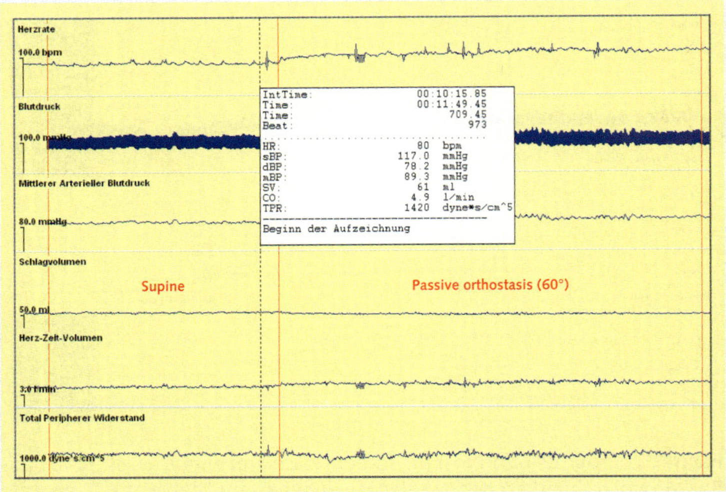

Figure 13 Initial situation before assuming the upright posture (for start of recording, see tool-tip box): heart rate 80 bpm, blood pressure 117/70 mmHg.

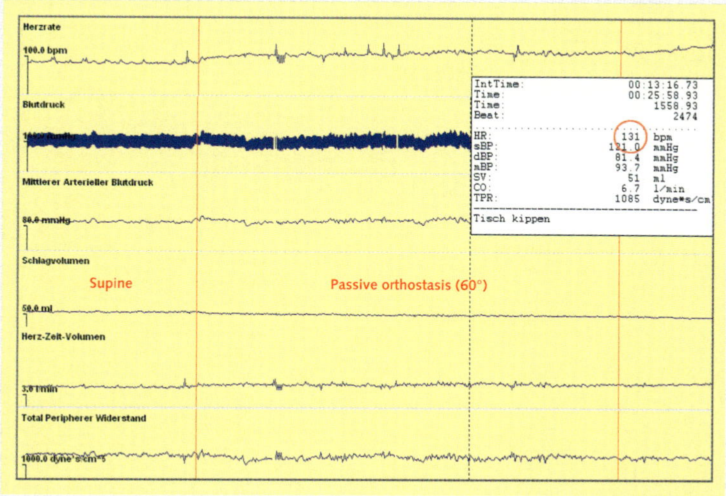

Figure 14 Progress of orthostatic response: 1. Heart rate rise of at least 30 bpm within 10 minutes after movement to the upright position, compared to baseline values when lying supine, 2. heart rate rise to at least 120 bpm (here 131 bpm (marker)), 3. no concurrent fall of systolic blood pressure by 20 mmHg or of diastolic blood pressure by 10 mmHg (here stable at 121/81 mmHg).
However, a specific diagnosis can only be established in concurrence with clinical symptoms of progressive orthostatic intolerance.

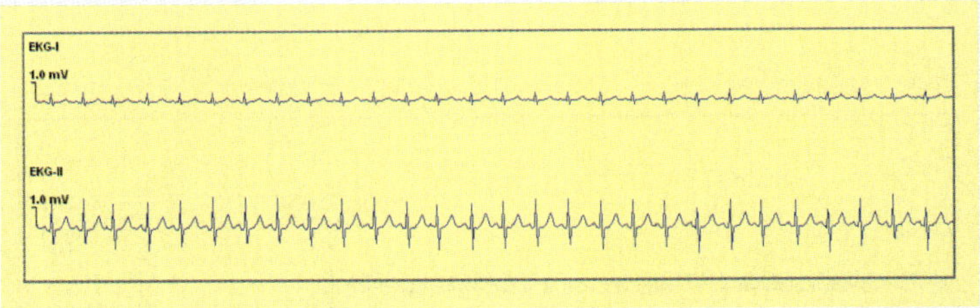

Figure 15 ECG signals during POTS and display of sinus tachycardia, HR-max 131/min.

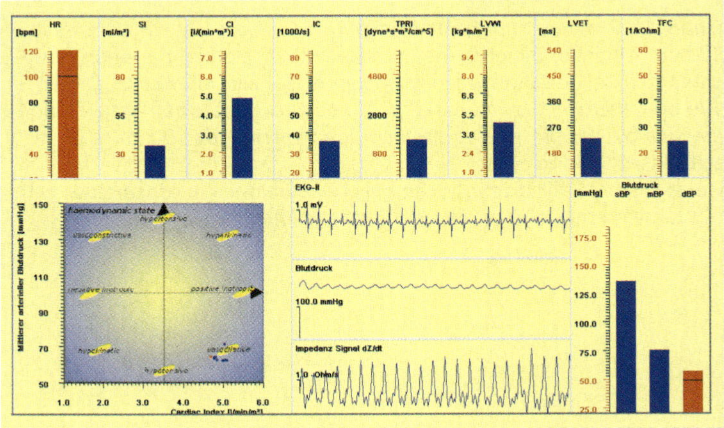

Figure 16 Cardiac parameters during POTS: tachycardia (HR, on the top left) with maintained blood pressure profile (at the bottom right), low total peripheral resistance index (TPRI, central on the top), low stroke index (SI, on the top left) and left ventricular index of contractility (IC), short left ventricular ejection time (LVET), and – due to tachycardia – normal cardiac index (CI).

2.2.2.3 Positive test result: carotid sinus syndrome

Table 9 Carotid sinus massage (protocol, test result)

Protocol
First exclusion of plaques and flow-limiting stenosis of carotid arteries by means of duplex ultrasonography, or at least auscultation of both carotid arteries. Application of equipment for continuous ECG and blood pressure recording. Undertaking of carotid sinus massage with the patient in both supine and upright positions: location of carotid sinus at the anterior margin of the sternocleidomastoid muscle at the level of the cricoid cartilage. At first, massage of the right carotid artery for a minimum of 5 and a maximum of 10 s; if no positive response occurs, massage of the left carotid artery.
Pathological test result • Asystole ≥ 3 s, and/or • fall of blood pressure ≥ 50 mmHg

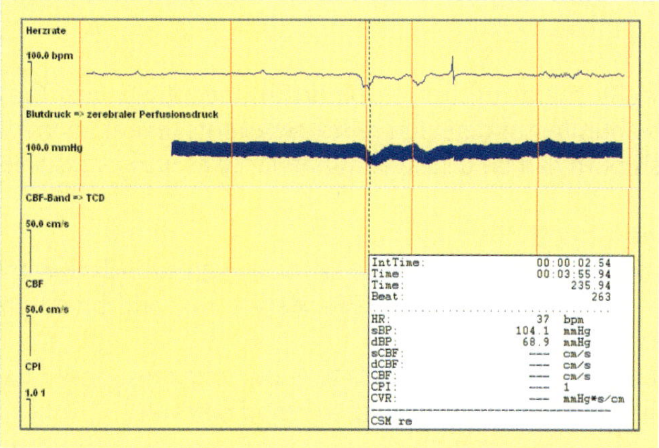

Figure 17 Overview of heart rate and blood pressure behavior during carotid sinus massage: reproducible bradycardias with a distinct fall in heart rate, and shortly afterwards also in blood pressure.

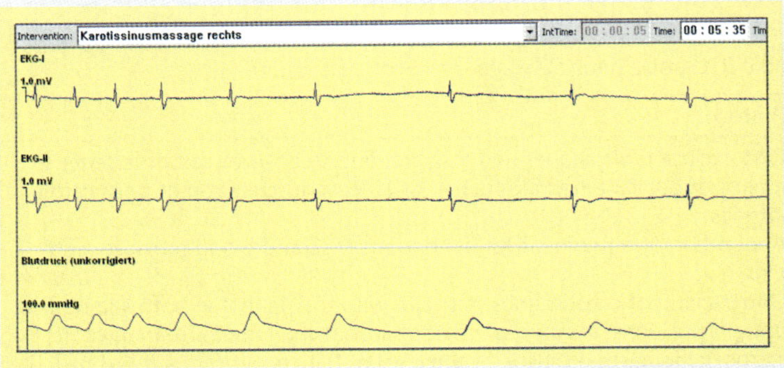

Figure 18 Bradycardia during carotid sinus massage with concurrent decline in blood pressure.

2.2.2.4 Baroreflex sensitivity: physiological and pathological behavior

Significant characteristics of baroreflex sensitivity are the slope and the number of detected reflex arc events (event count). In the analysis both can be displayed numerically as well as graphically.

a) Slope

The slope describes the steepness of a regression line within the coordinate axis of heart rate (RR-interval, ms) and blood pressure (mmHg).

A reduced slope corresponds to a low reflex response of a heart rate change following a change in blood pressure.

b) Event-count

The number of detected baroreceptor reflex events (event count) is related to one minute. A single event is registered by means of the spontaneous sequence method if consecutively disproportional changes occur within ≥ 3 subsequent heart beats: Either the blood pressure falls while the heart rate rises (up-event) or vice versa (down-event) (see Chapter 1.5.1).

The graphic illustration shows the regression lines of measured up- and down-events:

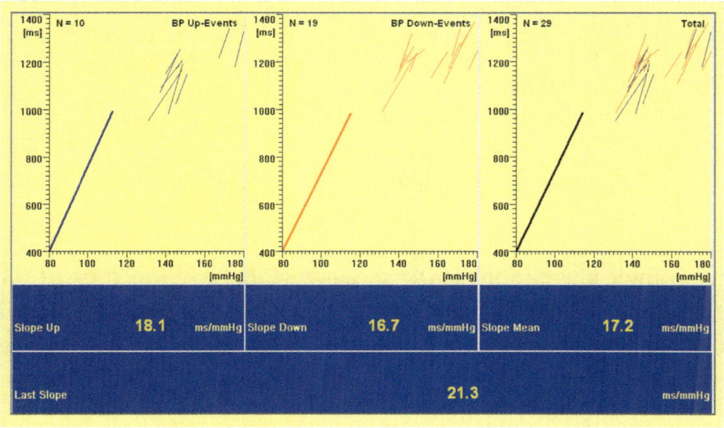

Figure 19 Normal values of baroreflex sensitivity: "down-events", i.e., fall in blood pressure and increase in heart rate (red), and vice versa "up-events" (blue). An event is displayed as a straight line whose steepness represents the amplitude of the respective reflex response. The regression line originating in the coordinate axis constitutes their mean value. Both the number of detected events (N) and the amplitude of the reflective responses (slope) are within the normal range.
In the case displayed: Normal number of detected baroreceptor reflex events (N = 29 within 10 min, i.e., 2.9/min) and normal amplitude of the reflective response (slope mean 17.2 ms/mmHg) for the age group of 18–29 years.

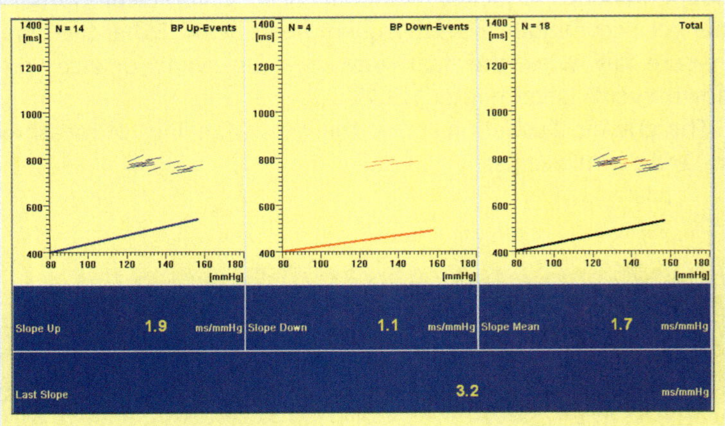

Figure 20 Pathological test result: normal number of detected baroreceptor reflex events (N = 18 within 10 min, i.e., 1.8/min), but considerably reduced amplitude of reflex response (slope mean 1.7 ms/mmHg) with shallow regression line.

2.2.2.5 Positive test result: impaired heart rate variability

The graphic illustration clearly shows a globally reduced heart rate variability, missing frequency ranges or a pathological withdrawal of single spectrum components before syncope.

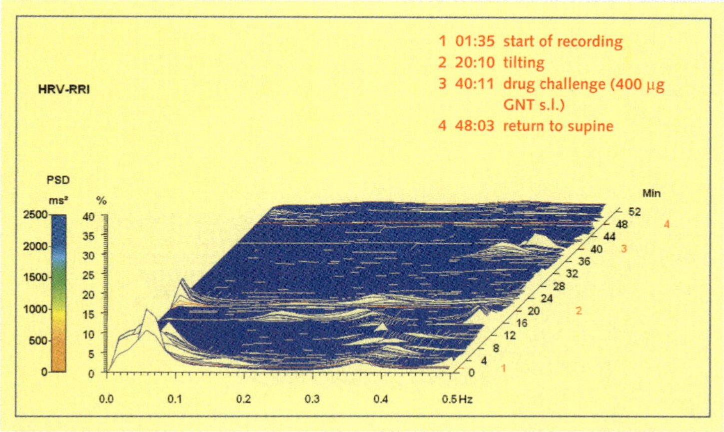

Figure 21 Virtually non-existent HRV within all frequency ranges in a patient with severe autonomic diabetic polyneuropathy, and missing response to orthostatic stress.

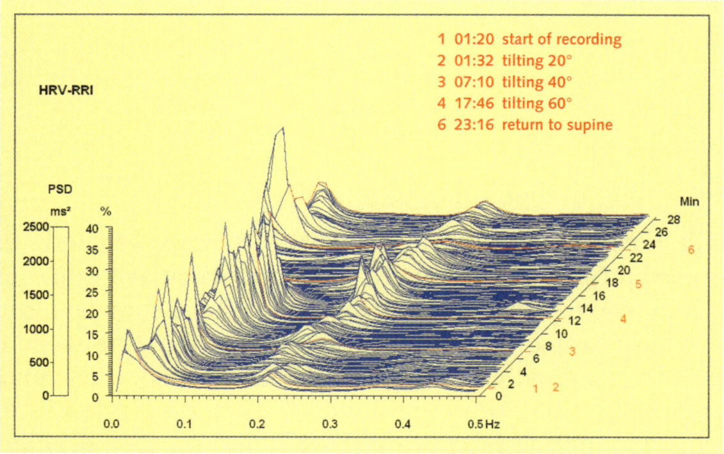

Figure 22 Autonomic diabetic polyneuropathy: low power spectral density in the LF-range, no modification of the frequency spectrum during passive orthostasis (a dominance of the LF-range and a reduction of the HF-range would be the physiological response to tilting).

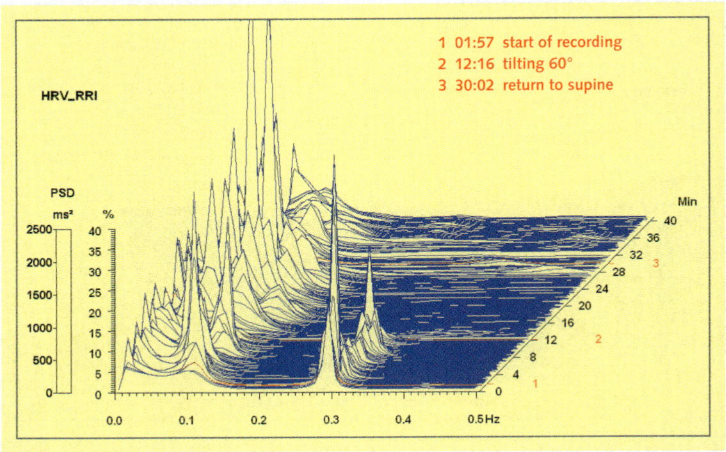

Figure 23 Withdrawal of vagal tone with disappearance of HF-range around 0.3 Hz and domination of sympathetic tone upon tilting, withdrawal of sympathetic tone after 30 minutes test duration, accompanied by onset of vasovagal syncope.

2.2.3 Tests of autonomic function

Aside from its application to the fields of syncope diagnosis, assessment of standard parameters of hemodynamic and cardiovascular autonomic functions, autonomic function testing by means of defined maneuvers is another example of the wide range of applications of non-invasive beat-to-beat monitoring. Autonomic function tests are particularly useful if there are indications for orthostatic intolerance associated with underlying autonomic dysfunctions associated with neurodegenerative diseases or diabetes mellitus (see Chapter 1.5.3).

The following tests are used in the selective or comprehensive evaluation of sympathetic and vagal functions:

a) Selective evaluation of the sympathetic system:

- *Sustained (isometric) handgrip test*

This pressor test generates a stimulation of the sympathetic efferent fibers that is independent of baroreceptor afference.

Table 10 Sustained handgrip test (protocol, normal value)

Protocol
A hand-dynamometer or a partly inflated blood pressure cuff is compressed with a handgrip of about 30%.
Normal value: rise in diastolic blood pressure by ≥ 16 mmHg.

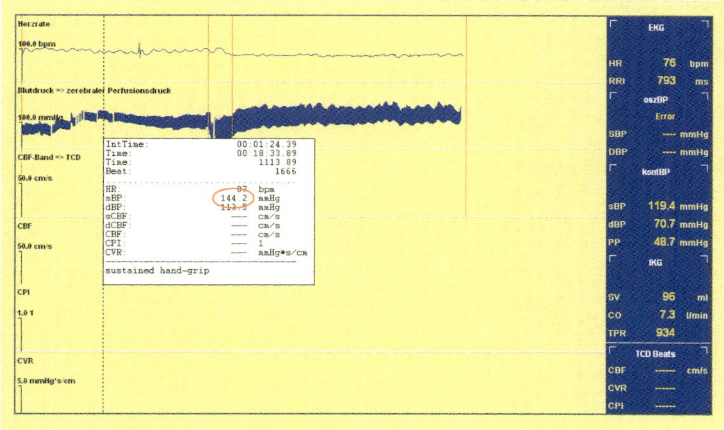

Figure 24 Normal response of the sympathetic efferent system, resulting in a blood pressure rise from 121 mmHg to 144 mmHg (marker) during isometric handgrip.

b) Selective evaluation of the vagal system:

- *Heart rate variability during deep breathing (E/I-difference and E/I-ratio)*

The evaluation of heart rate variability during deep breathing shows physiological responses that consist of an increased heart rate during inspiration and of a decline in heart rate during expiration, which is mediated chiefly by changing vagal activity.

Table 11 E/I-difference, E/I-ratio (protocol, normal values)

Protocol	
The subject is sitting and is told to breathe deeply and regularly with 6 breaths per minute, i.e., with inspiration and expiration phases of 5 s each. (It is recommended that the test is < 2 minutes, otherwise resulting hypocapnia accounts for increased heart rate and reduced heart rate variability.) This test allows the calculation of the following parameters: a) the E/I-difference, which results from the difference between the highest and the lowest heart rate values obtained during the examination period, and b) the E/I-ratio, which represents the quotient from the longest over the shortest RR-intervals obtained during the examination period.	
Normal values – E/I-difference (bpm)	**Age (years)**
18	10–40
16	41–50
12	51–60
8	61–70
Normal values – E/I-ratio	
1.24	< 15
1.23	16–20
1.20	21–25
1.18	26–30
1.16	31–35
1.14	36–40
1.12	41–45
1.11	46–50
1.09	51–55
1.08	56–60
1.07	61–65
1.06	66–70
1.06	71–75

Intervention: Inspiration/Exspirationsmanöver IntTime: 00 : 00 : 00 Time: 00 : 10 : 35 Time: 635.10

Beschreibung	RRI [ms]	HR [bpm]	sBP [mmHg]	dBP [mmHg]	mBP [mmHg]	SV [ml]	SI [ml/m²]	CO [l/min]	CI [l/(min*m²)]	TPR [dyne*s/cm^5]	TPRI [dyne*s*m²/cm^5]
Beginn der Aufzeichnung											
N	397	397	397	397	397	397	397	397	397	397	397
Min	608	75.1	139.5	91.2	106.9	66	27.7	5.0	2.1	878	2095
Max	799	98.6	164.5	124.8	134.7	107	44.8	10.2	4.3	1899	4532
Mean	743	80.9	149.7	101.3	118.1	78	32.9	6.4	2.7	1469	3505
SD	25	2.9	5.0	4.2	4.7	7	3.1	0.7	0.3	169	404
SEM	1.25	0.14	0.25	0.21	0.24	0.37	0.16	0.04	0.02	8.49	20.25
Orthostase											
N	336	336	336	336	336	333	333	333	333	333	333
Min	575	69.1	132.8	92.4	106.0	51	21.6	4.2	1.8	941	2244
Max	869	104.4	204.7	135.7	156.1	106	44.3	11.0	4.6	2843	6784
Mean	680	88.6	162.3	111.5	128.9	73	30.6	6.5	2.7	1576	3762
SD	44	5.7	13.8	10.0	11.3	7	3.0	0.8	0.3	234	559
SEM	2.42	0.31	0.75	0.54	0.61	0.40	0.17	0.05	0.02	12.83	30.62
Inspiration/Exspirationsm											
N	143	143	143	143	143	141	141	141	141	141	141
Min	538	88.1	104.7	68.1	84.6	68	28.4	6.5	2.7	815	1946
Max	681	111.6	184.7	118.9	146.3	86	36.0	9.3	3.9	1573	3755
Mean	603	99.9	138.8	92.1	111.5	77	32.4	7.7	3.2	1138	2715
SD	35	5.9	21.7	12.0	15.6	4	1.7	0.6	0.3	210	501
SEM	2.95	0.49	1.81	1.00	1.31	0.33	0.14	0.05	0.02	17.69	42.20

Figure 25 Data view of an autonomic function test: shortest RR-interval 538 ms, longest RR-interval 681 ms during inspiration (marker), corresponding to an E/I-ratio of 1.27. Maximum HR 112 bpm, minimum HR 88 bpm, corresponding to an E/I-difference of 24 bpm.

- *Active orthostasis (30:15 ratio, age-related)*

Upon standing venous pooling in the lower extremities occurs and causes a transient decline in cardiac preload and stroke volume. Due to rapid compensatory measures there are only slight changes in arterial blood pressure in healthy subjects.

Heart rate fluctuations occurring within the first 30 (40) seconds after moving to the upright posture allow an evaluation of the cardiovagal system, defined as the "30:15"-ratio or "Ewing-ratio", describing an age-related reproducible index.

In the setting of diagnosing orthostatic disorders, a decrease in systolic blood pressure of at least 20 mmHg or a decrease in diastolic blood pressure of at least 10 mmHg within three minutes after standing up are diagnostic indications for orthostatic intolerance, a condition that has to be differentiated from vasovagal syncope (see Chapter 1.2.3.3).

If orthostatic symptoms are so pronounced that the subject does not tolerate standing for at least three minutes, the "standing-time" until the onset of orthostatic symptoms is noted as well.

Table 12 30:15-ratio (protocol, normal values)

Protocol	
The preparatory phase comprises the application of equipment for ECG and non-invasive blood pressure recording and an equilibration period of 5–10 minutes with the patient in supine position. Then the patient assumes the upright posture while breathing calmly and regularly. The 30:15-ratio is obtained by calculating the quotient from the longest RR-interval between the 20th and the 40th heart beat over the shortest RR-interval between the 5th and the 25th heart beat after standing up.	
Normal values 30:15-ratio	**Age (years)**
1.20	< 15
1.18	16–20
1.17	21–25
1.15	26–30
1.13	31–35
1.11	36–40
1.09	41–45
1.08	46–50
1.06	51–55
1.04	56–60
1.02	61–65
1.01	66–70
1.0	71–75

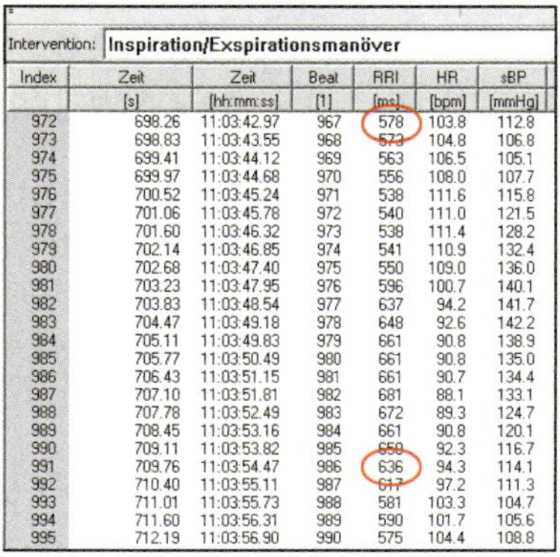

Intervention: Inspiration/Exspirationsmanöver

Index	Zeit [s]	Zeit [hh:mm:ss]	Beat [1]	RRI [ms]	HR [bpm]	sBP [mmHg]
972	698.26	11:03:42.97	967	578	103.8	112.8
973	698.83	11:03:43.55	968	573	104.8	106.8
974	699.41	11:03:44.12	969	563	106.5	105.1
975	699.97	11:03:44.68	970	556	108.0	107.7
976	700.52	11:03:45.24	971	538	111.6	115.8
977	701.06	11:03:45.78	972	540	111.0	121.5
978	701.60	11:03:46.32	973	538	111.4	128.2
979	702.14	11:03:46.85	974	541	110.9	132.4
980	702.68	11:03:47.40	975	550	109.0	136.0
981	703.23	11:03:47.95	976	596	100.7	140.1
982	703.83	11:03:48.54	977	637	94.2	141.7
983	704.47	11:03:49.18	978	648	92.6	142.2
984	705.11	11:03:49.83	979	661	90.8	138.9
985	705.77	11:03:50.49	980	661	90.8	135.0
986	706.43	11:03:51.15	981	661	90.7	134.4
987	707.10	11:03:51.81	982	681	88.1	133.1
988	707.78	11:03:52.49	983	672	89.3	124.7
989	708.45	11:03:53.16	984	661	90.8	120.1
990	709.11	11:03:53.82	985	650	92.3	116.7
991	709.76	11:03:54.47	986	636	94.3	114.1
992	710.40	11:03:55.11	987	617	97.2	111.3
993	711.01	11:03:55.73	988	581	103.3	104.7
994	711.60	11:03:56.31	989	590	101.7	105.6
995	712.19	11:03:56.90	990	575	104.4	108.8

Figure 26 Calculation of 30:15-ratio by the shortest and longest RR-intervals within the 5th and the 40th heart beats (markers) after assumption of upright posture. In this case the 20th beat and the 5th beat result in a 30:15-ratio of 1.18.

c) Comprehensive evaluation of sympathetic and vagal functions

- *Valsalva maneuver*

The response of the cardiovascular system to this maneuver provides insights into the cardiovascular sympathetic and vagal system and also into the function of the baroreceptor reflex.

The response can be divided into four phases (see Chapter 1.5.3.3). The Valsalva-ratio, as a measure of heart rate variations during the Valsalva maneuver, is considered as an established index for evaluating the function of the vagal system.

Table 13 Valsalva-ratio (protocol, normal values)

Protocol	
The patient is sitting and generates an intrathoracic pressure rise of ~40 mmHg during cycles of 15 s by means of continuous forcible exhalation, e.g., against a special mouthpiece. For a reliable interpretation of the results the maneuver should be repeated three times. The Valsalva-ratio is calculated by the quotient from the longest RR-interval after the maneuver over the shortest interval during or shortly after the maneuver.	
Normal values – Valsalva-ratio	**Age (years)**
1.53	< 15
1.48	16–20
1.43	21–25
1.38	26–30
1.33	31–35
1.28	36–40
1.24	41–45
1.20	46–50
1.16	51–55
1.12	56–60
1.08	61–65
1.04	66–70
1.0	71–75

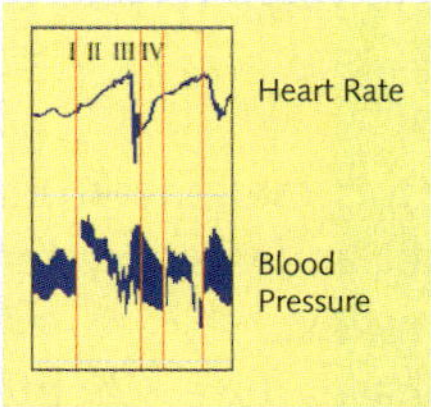

Figure 27 High-resolution display of the various phases during a Valsalva maneuver:
Phase I: short drop in HR for a few seconds, increase in blood pressure. Phase IIa: decline in blood pressure. Phase IIb: increase in heart rate. Phase III: further decline in blood pressure. Phase IV: abrupt increase in blood pressure and fall in heart rate.

Table 14 Physiological and pathological changes during the various phases of a Valsalva maneuver

Disturbance	Phase I	Phase II (early)	Phase II (late)	Phase III	Phase IV
No disturbance	Stress-dependent rise in blood pressure	Decrease in arterial blood pressure	Increase in arterial blood pressure	Short-term decrease in blood pressure	Exaggerated rise in blood pressure
Vagal disturbance	Normal reaction	Reduced decline in blood pressure	Normal reaction	Normal reaction	Normal reaction
Slight sympathetic disturbance	Normal reaction	Slightly more pronounced decrease in blood pressure	Reduced or missing increase in blood pressure	Normal reaction	Slight reduction in the increase in blood pressure
Moderate sympathetic disturbance	Normal reaction	Highly developed decrease in blood pressure	Missing increase in blood pressure	Normal reaction	Distinctly less pronounced rise in blood pressure
Severe sympathetic disturbance	Normal reaction	Extremely developed decrease in blood pressure	Missing increase in blood pressure	Normal reaction	Missing increase in blood pressure

By means of continuous blood pressure and heart rate monitoring it is possible to analyze occurring changes during the phases of a Valsalva maneuver and to draw conclusions as to the diagnosis and degree of dysfunctions (see Table 14) [335].

2.2.4 Cardiac pacemaker therapy

The combination of impedance cardiography and non-invasive blood pressure monitoring enables the identification of diagnostic markers for cardiac contractility. These are subject to changes due to dual chamber cardiac pacemaker resettings, e.g., by programming optimal AV-delays or by optimizing the synchronous function of cardiac resynchronization therapy devices. In this setting the following parameters carry great weight (for explanations, see Chapter 2.2.1):

- Systolic blood pressure (mmHg)
- Stroke volume (ml) and stroke index (ml/m²)
- Cardiac output (L/min) and cardiac index (L/min/m²)
- Index of contractility (1/1000 s)
- Acceleration index (1/100 s²)
- Maximum rise in pressure [dP/dt_{max}] (mmHg/s)

The influence of reprogrammed dual chamber cardiac pacemakers or resynchronization devices on the behavior of stroke volume and blood pressure can be displayed both in tabular form and in continuous real time graphics.

After applying the measurement devices (ECG, impedance cardiography, non-invasive blood pressure monitoring) to the patient it is recommended that one minute is waited between each reprogramming of the PM/CRT-systems so that the program change can begin to take hemodynamic effect and therefore to become discernible.

A change of contractility parameters can be displayed either graphically or in the data view (Fig. 30).

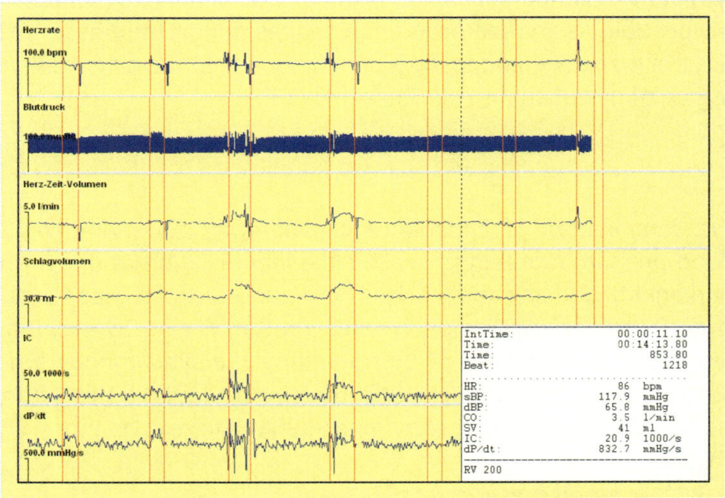

Figure 28 Left ventricular parameters during CRT-optimization. Graphic illustration of the behavior of heart rate (HR), blood pressure (sBP, dBP), stroke volume (SV), index of contractility (IC) and of left ventricular contractility (dP/dt). In the "tool-tip box" parameter values (including cardiac output [CO]) are displayed at the chosen moment.

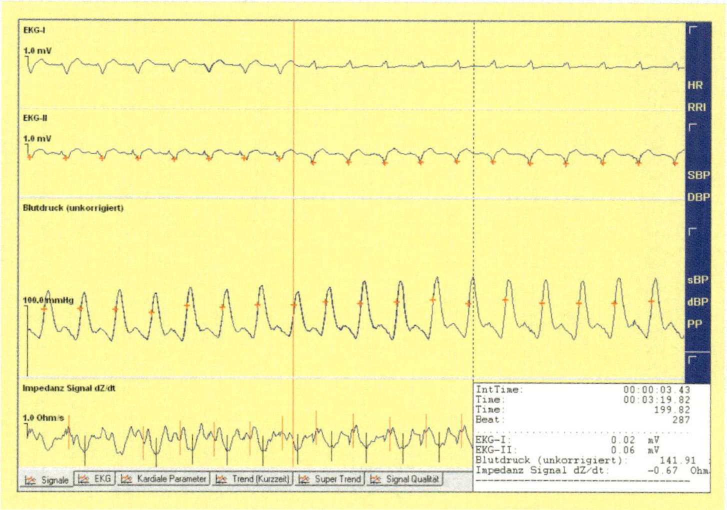

Figure 29 Blood pressure change after CRT-optimization. The QRS-enlargement displayed in the surface-ECG is declining, the blood pressure amplitude is rising, the impedance cardiography signal during systole is becoming increasingly monophasic.

Intervention: AV III IntTime:

Index	Zeit [s]	Zeit [hh:mm:ss]	Beat [1]	RRI [ms]	HR [bpm]	sBP [mmHg]	dBP [mmHg]	mBP [mmHg]	SV [ml]	SI [ml/m²]	CO [l/min]
483	487.00	10:49:08.75	475	1186	50.6	124.2	75.9	91.8	65	35.4	3.3
484	488.18	10:49:09.94	476	1148	52.3	121.2	77.0	90.9	62	33.8	3.3
485	489.33	10:49:11.09	477	1224	49.0	125.5	75.1	92.9	62	33.8	3.1
486	490.55	10:49:12.31	478	1209	49.6	121.8	75.2	90.6	63	34.4	3.1
487	491.76	10:49:13.52	479	1196	50.2	122.1	75.8	90.6	60	32.6	3.0
488	492.96	10:49:14.72	480	1235	48.6	124.1	74.8	91.2	62	33.7	3.0
489	494.19	10:49:15.95	481	1221	49.1	122.4	75.3	90.0	67	36.5	3.3
490	495.42	10:49:17.17	482	1177	51.0	122.2	75.6	90.1	64	34.8	3.3
491	496.59	10:49:18.35	483	1207	49.7	122.3	74.5	90.2	63	34.5	3.2
492	497.80	10:49:19.56	484	1144	52.4	122.4	76.3	90.1	63	34.3	3.3
493	498.94	10:49:20.70	485	1079	55.6	122.3	77.9	91.6	62	33.7	3.5
494	500.02	10:49:21.78	486	1127	53.2	125.1	80.0	94.7	59	32.3	3.2
495	501.15	10:49:22.91	487	1109	54.1	120.9	77.7	92.7	60	32.6	3.2
496	502.26	10:49:24.01	488	1159	51.8	124.0	79.9	95.0	62	34.0	3.2
497	503.42	10:49:25.17	489	1161	51.7	125.2	77.3	93.9	64	34.5	3.3
498	504.58	10:49:26.33	490	1134	52.9	123.9	78.0	93.2	58	31.4	3.1
499	505.71	10:49:27.47	491	1166	51.5	124.2	74.9	91.8	57	31.0	2.9
500	506.88	10:49:28.63	492	1155	51.9	122.6	74.7	90.1	58	31.4	3.0
501	508.03	10:49:29.79	493	1125	53.3	121.2	73.3	88.7	55	29.9	2.9
502	509.16	10:49:30.91	494	1133	53.0	121.5	73.2	88.6	56	30.6	3.0
503	510.29	10:49:32.05	495	1129	53.1	119.6	71.4	86.9	59	32.0	3.1
504	511.42	10:49:33.18	496	1676	35.8	120.1	72.2	88.1	60	32.8	2.2
505	512.30	10:51:07.76	DTD 7(	======	======	======	======	======	======	======	======
506	513.09	10:51:08.55	497	859	69.8	118.5	70.7	83.5	72	38.9	5.0
507	513.95	10:51:09.41	498	858	69.9	116.1	69.5	82.2	74	40.3	5.2
508	514.81	10:51:10.27	499	861	69.7	117.7	70.5	82.9	84	45.5	5.8
509	515.67	10:51:11.13	500	854	70.2	117.8	70.5	83.4	83	45.3	5.9
510	516.53	10:51:11.99	501	859	69.8	116.0	69.5	82.1	76	41.4	5.3
511	517.39	10:51:12.85	502	857	70.0	117.7	70.4	82.9	75	41.0	5.3
512	518.24	10:51:13.70	503	859	69.9	117.9	69.5	83.0	---	---	---
513	519.10	10:51:14.56	504	865	69.4	115.9	68.9	81.7	80	43.7	5.6
514	519.97	10:51:15.43	505	858	69.9	117.7	69.9	82.6	80	43.6	5.6
515	520.83	10:51:16.29	506	860	69.8	117.3	69.3	82.3	86	46.8	6.0
516	521.69	10:51:17.15	507	858	70.0	115.2	68.6	81.1	87	47.3	6.1
517	522.54	10:51:18.00	508	858	69.9	117.0	69.6	82.0	96	52.1	6.7
518	523.40	10:51:18.86	509	859	69.9	114.8	68.6	81.2	92	50.2	6.5

Figure 30 Increase in stroke volume (SV, marker), in a comparison between 3rd degree AV-block and dual chamber stimulation displayed in tabular form.

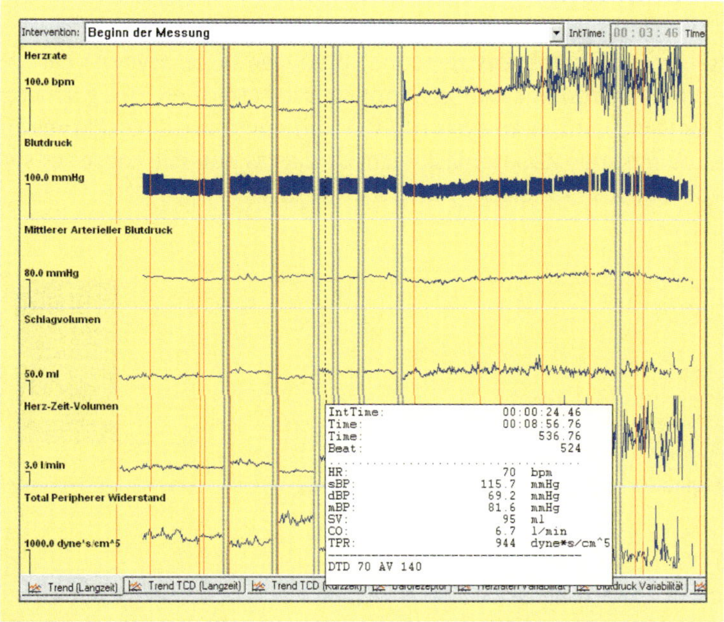

Figure 31 Graphic illustration of blood pressure and stroke volume during program changes of a dual chamber cardiac pacemaker. Artefacts occurring during the last examination phase are caused by stress testing (bicycle ergometry with applied measuring electrodes).

2.2.5 Rhythm analysis

During cardioinhibitory syncope, bradycardia or asystole can occur regularly during examinations. In the case of recurring syncope or presyncope the analysis of ECG and continuous blood pressure recordings may also unmask tachycardias as possible causes of syncope (see also Chapter 3, case 4).

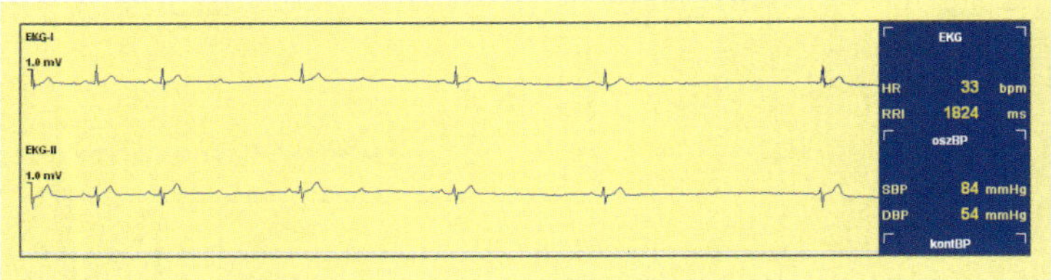

Figure 32 Detection of 2nd degree AV block.

3 Case studies

Case 1 Vasovagal syncope – VASIS IIb

Medical history:
Male patient, 37 years, within the last three years three documented losses of consciousness, two of them in association with venepuncture and one during physiotherapy of shoulder impingement syndrome. No past medical history or family history of other diseases.

Suspected diagnosis:
Vasovagal, situational (pain-induced) syncope.

Procedure:
No further diagnostic assessment necessary. At the patient's specific request exploration by tilt table testing was performed (Fig. 33).

Diagnosis:
Vasovagal syncope, cardioinhibitory form with asystole (VASIS IIb).

Commentary and therapy:
The symptoms corresponded completely with the episodes of loss of consciousness that occurred during ambulatory testing. The diagnosis of vasovagal syncope is confirmed.

The low frequency of syncopal events, the fact that the patient does not belong to a high-risk group and the clear triggering event are factors that do not warrant further therapeutic measures. Situations associated with painful stimuli should be avoided as much as possible, withdrawal of blood should be accompanied by a prolonged supine phase.

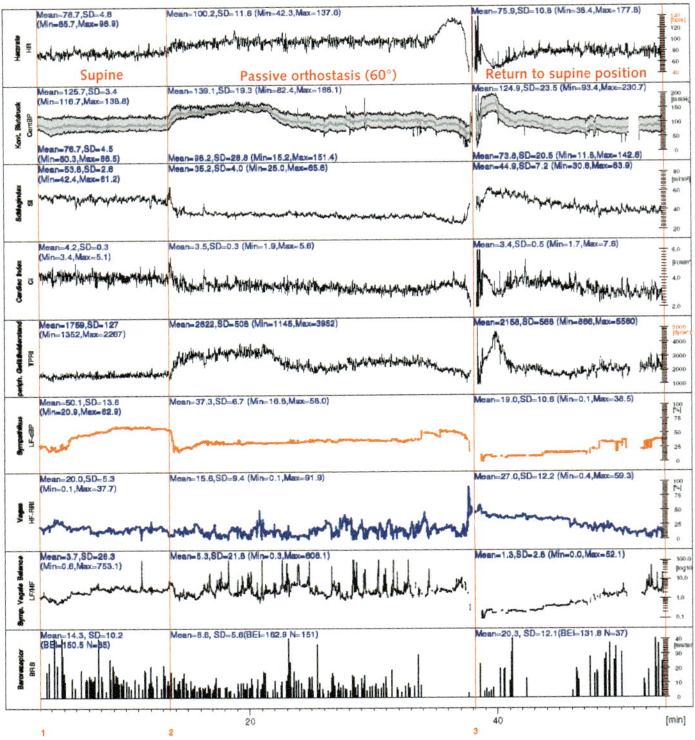

Figure 33 1-page-diagnosis-report of the Task Force Monitor.
Marker 1: start of recording, marker 2: tilting to 60°, marker 3: resetting of table to supine position upon onset of syncope after 24 minutes of passive orthostasis.
The following events can be detected (from top to bottom): 1. fall in heart rate after presyncopal increase; 2. concurrent decrease in blood pressure; 3. decrease of stroke volume index and cardiac index during upright posture; 4. increase and subsequent progressive decrease of peripheral resistance; 5. withdrawal of sympathetic tone prior to onset of syncope; 6. increase of sympatho-vagal balance during standing and inversion of ratio during syncope; 7. reduction of baroreflex sensitivity prior to and during syncope. Another pathological feature is the more or less constant high frequency component of heart rate (HF-RRI) and the initial decrease after assuming the upright position of low frequency component of diastolic blood pressure (LF-dBP).

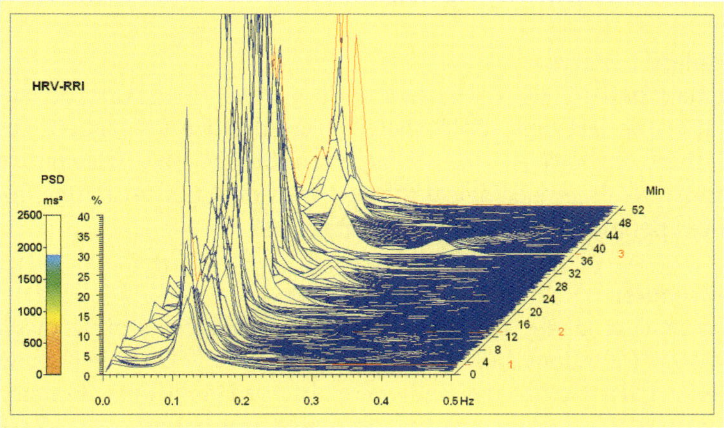

Figure 34 Three-dimensional illustration of the development of heart rate variability in the patient mentioned above: sudden withdrawal of sympathetic tone with temporary disappearance of LF-range and onset of vasovagal syncope. Slow recovery of LF-range after table has been tilted back. During syncope sudden dominance of HF-signal.

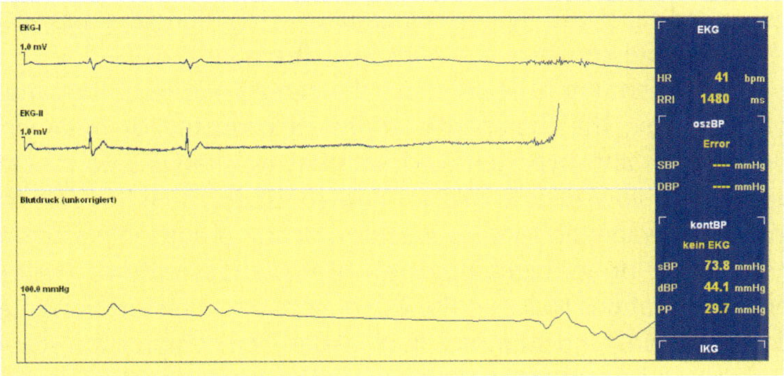

Figure 35 High resolution ECG at the time of syncope: display of start of asystole, which lasted a total of 32 s.

Case 2 Vasovagal syncope – VASIS III

Medical history:
Female patient, 60 years, two episodes of loss of consciousness within the last year. Both spells occurred while the patient was washing the dishes. Arterial hypertension the only relevant comorbidity. Pharmacological therapy with diuretics, ACE-inhibitors and a peripheral alpha-receptor antagonist.

Procedure:
The analysis of the questionnaire yielded indications of vasovagal syncope (questions 1, 3, 6 answered with "yes"). Discrete negative T waves in the precordial leads were observed in the initial examination, and so echocardiography (left ventricular hypertrophy 12 mm septal, 13 mm posterior) and an exercise-test (as to ischemic repolarization disorders inconspicuous until 150 watts) were performed in parallel. On account of the medical history obtained by the questionnaire a tilt table test was performed (see Fig. 36).

Suspected diagnosis:
Vasovagal syncope.

Commentary and therapy:
The symptoms that were reproduced during tilt table testing corresponded exactly to those documented, establishing the diagnosis of "vasodepressor vasovagal syncope" (VASIS III).

After patient information about the benign nature of the symptom complex, the therapeutic approach consisted of modifying the patient's anti-hypertensive treatment by changing to a beta-blocker and slow-release calcium-antagonist drugs. In this case the ensuing therapeutic success was not clearly predictable since all hypertensive drugs might aggravate orthostatic symptoms. Further recommendations included the use of compression stockings, regular tilt training and sufficient fluid intake. The compression stockings should be custom-made to meet the requirement of a minimum pressure of 30–40 mmHg in the malleolar region. Prolonged standing is to be avoided. If a syncopal attack occurs the patient

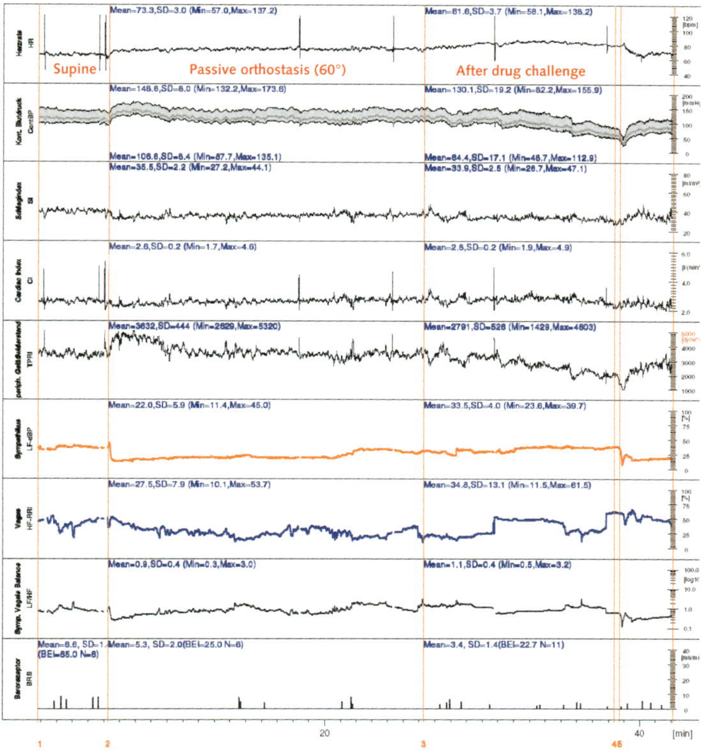

Figure 36 1-page-diagnosis-report of the Task Force Monitor.
The following events can be detected (from top to bottom): 1. stable to increasing heart rate; 2. progressive decline in blood pressure until onset of syncope after 33 minutes of passive tilting or 13 minutes after drug challenge (400 µg GTN sl.), respectively; 3. slight decrease of stroke volume index and cardiac index during standing; 4. increase and subsequent progressive decrease in peripheral resistance; 5. withdrawal of sympathetic tone upon onset of syncope.
Further pathological test results are a) the decreasing low frequency component of diastolic blood pressure (LF-dBP), b) the impaired baroreflex sensitivity in supine and upright postures concerning this age group (female, 60 years) (upright posture: slope 6.8 ms/mmHg, 6 events/5 minutes = 1.2/min; normal value: slope 7.3 ms/mmHg, event-count 1.7/min).

should assume a supine position and, if possible, perform isometric counterpressure maneuvers of the arms or quick leg-crossing.

Vasodepressor forms of orthostatic intolerance also occur notably in the setting of severe autonomic dysfunctions (see Table 5) and should be excluded by means of medical history taking and clinical examinations.

Case 3 Presyncope: POTS

Medical history:
Female patient, 23 years, reported being highly afflicted and troubled by vertigo, nausea, visual disturbances and anxiety during prolonged standing, as well as by a feeling of constant fatigue and stress intolerance. No loss of consciousness so far, no relevant comorbidities.

Procedure:
The questionnaire was inconclusive, the basic evaluation did not reveal any abnormalities. Tilt table testing was performed to reproduce the reported symptoms (Fig. 37).

Suspected diagnosis:
Orthostatic intolerance.

Commentary and therapy:
Controlled upright tilt table testing produced tachycardia, vertigo, diplopia and nausea, thus reproducing the perceived symptoms and establishing the diagnosis of "postural orthostatic tachycardia syndrome".

First, the patient was informed about the benign nature of the symptom complex. Since incapacitating orthostatic symptoms continued to occur in spite of the reassurance regarding the harmless nature of the condition, further therapeutic measures consisted of prescribing a serotonin reuptake inhibitor (20 mg paroxetine), and the patient was recommended to ensure sufficient fluid intake and to avoid alcohol consumption. Moderate aerobic exercise at least three times a week was also recommended.

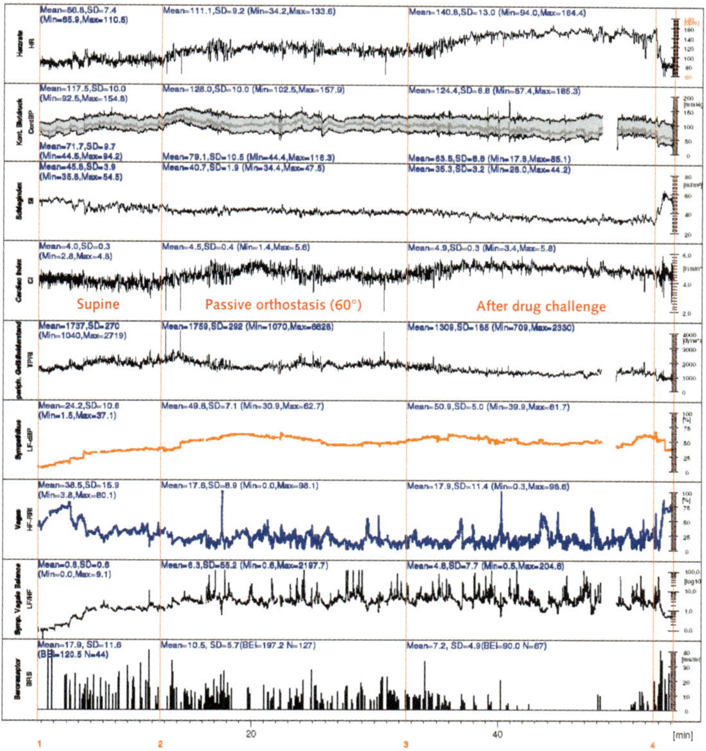

Figure 37 1-page-diagnosis-report of the Task Force Monitor.
The following events can be detected (from top to bottom): 1. progressively increasing heart rate from a mean baseline value of ~87 bpm to a mean 140 bpm during standing, with an upward trend; 2. stable blood pressure behavior; 3. declining stroke volume, and – due to tachycardia – increasing cardiac index during upright position; 4. decrease of peripheral resistance; 5. permanent prevalence of sympathetic activity within the frequency spectrum of diastolic blood pressure withdrawal; 6. reduced heart rate regulating activity of parasympathetic component and subsequently increased sympatho-vagal balance; 7. reduction of baroreflex sensitivity during tachycardia.

Case 4 Presyncope: Paroxysmal atrial fibrillation

Medical history:
Female patient, 74 years, with position-independent attacks of vertigo several times a day, including palpitations and a feeling of imminent loss of consciousness. Relevant co-morbidities are: coronary heart disease (without any flow-limiting coronary stenosis) diagnosed by means of coronary angiography, well regulated arterial hypertension and chronic venous insufficiency.

Procedure:
The basic evaluation was inconclusive, the questionnaire was not used. With regard to a suspected orthostatic component correlated with chronic venous insufficiency, tilt table testing, Holter ECG monitoring and echocardiography were performed to diagnose and differentiate the reported complaints.

Suspected diagnosis:
Unclear recurring presyncope.

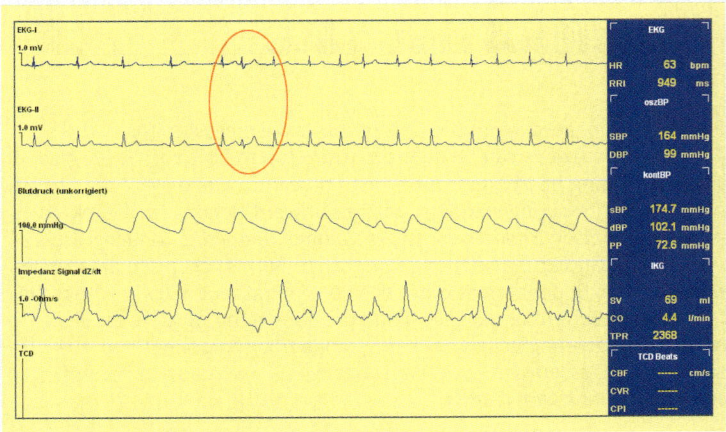

Figure 38 Induction of atrial fibrillation by a premature atrial contraction with concurrent reduction of blood pressure amplitude.

Commentary and therapy:

The analysis of long-term rhythm trends during tilt table testing showed several phases of intermittent tachycardias, while concurrent blood pressure monitoring documented a fall in blood pressure upon the onset of atrial fibrillation, thus correlating with the patient's complaints.

Beta-blocker therapy did not produce the desired anti-arrhythmic effect, in all probability the triggering mechanism actually consisted of bradycardia with a prolonged atrial repolarization phase and a subsequent vulnerability to supraventricular premature contractions. Because of the patient's highly restricted quality of life due to the reccurring symptoms, she underwent implantation of a dual chamber cardiac pacemaker with anti-tachycardiac atrial detection and stimulation algorithms.

Case 5 Orthostatic syncope: Shy-Drager syndrome

Medical history:

Male patient, 57 years, with progressively increasing recurrences of vertigo and loss of consciousness with falling, especially upon change from sitting to standing posture, ~30 minutes after meals and after nocturnal urination. Co-morbidities are: chronic constipation, many years of needing to urinate several times per night, as well as sexual impotency.

Procedure:

Neurological evaluation revealed mild dysarthria, slight stiffness of hands and neck, and – regarding the patient's gait – markedly small steps. In addition to the initial evaluation being inconclusive, the questionnaire was not suggestive.

Tilt table testing was performed among others to diagnose and differentiate the reported complaints (Fig. 39).

Suspected diagnosis:

Suspected orthostatic intolerance due to multiple system atrophy.

Commentary and therapy:
The clinical presentation describes symptoms of multiple system atrophy with pronounced orthostatic intolerance and – less prominent and having occurred at a later stage of the disease – Parkinsonian symptoms.

Clinical findings suggest a diagnosis of "multiple system atrophy with prevalent autonomic dysfunction and orthostatic intolerance (Shy-Drager syndrome)".

Multiple system atrophy may also manifest as so-called olivopontocerebellar atrophy, when associated with cerebellar symptoms (i.e., ataxia, dysathria), or as striatonigral degeneration, when associated with a prevalent presentation of Parkinsonian symptoms. Differentiation from Parkinson's disease with its typical clinical manifestations or from pure autonomic failure with its isolated deficits of the autonomic nervous system is difficult, especially in the early stages [187,209].

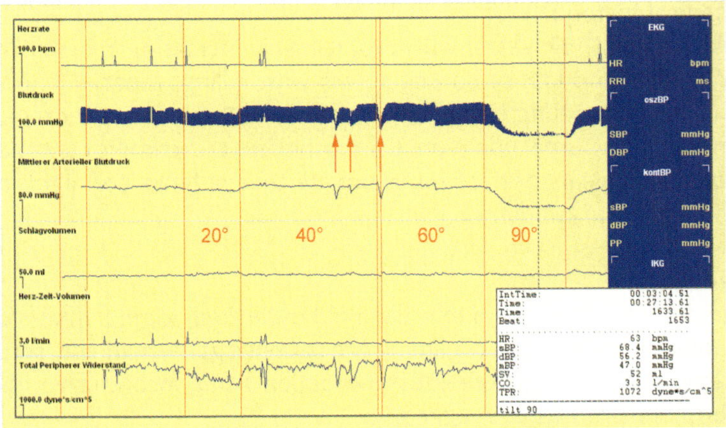

Figure 39 Survey of tilt table test procedure. The chosen protocol included a tilt angle increased progressively from 20–40–60 to 90°. Notable are: 1. missing response of heart rate; 2. recurring spontaneous drops in blood pressure (arrows); and 3. extremely developed orthostatic hypotension with stable heart rate during tilting at 90° until the end of the test.

Therapeutic measures consisted of prescription of an alpha-mimetic agent and recommendation of sufficient fluid and salt intake. Aggravating dysuria due to peripheral alpha-agonist medication became problematic. Cystometry revealed a declining compliance of the urinary bladder with detrusor-sphincter dyssynergia. Over time the patient learned to perform intermittent self-catheterization.

Where the disease is rapidly progressive, levodopa treatment may relieve symptoms, but the potential to concurrently aggravate orthostatic symptoms must be expected.

Case 6 Syncope: Carotid sinus hypersensitivity

Medical history:
Male patient, 86 years, with a history of recurrent falls, known diabetes mellitus, insulin-dependent. Other co-morbidities are: chronic obstructive pulmonary disease and gastric ulcer. A home care nurse found the patient unconscious, and the alerted emergency physician diagnosed an elevated blood glucose level with hyperosmolar diabetic coma. In the intensive care unit a central venous catheter was inserted into the right jugular vein. During palpitation of the carotid artery recurrent falls in heart rate were observed.

Suspected diagnosis:
Carotid sinus hypersensitivity.

Procedure:
In order to reproduce clinical features, heart rate and continuous non-invasive blood pressure monitoring were documented (Fig. 40).

Commentary and therapy:
The patient reported having suffered vertigo and a graying-out of vision for a long time, particularly upon head rotation. Home care nurses reported observing vertigo and presyncope also during shaving.

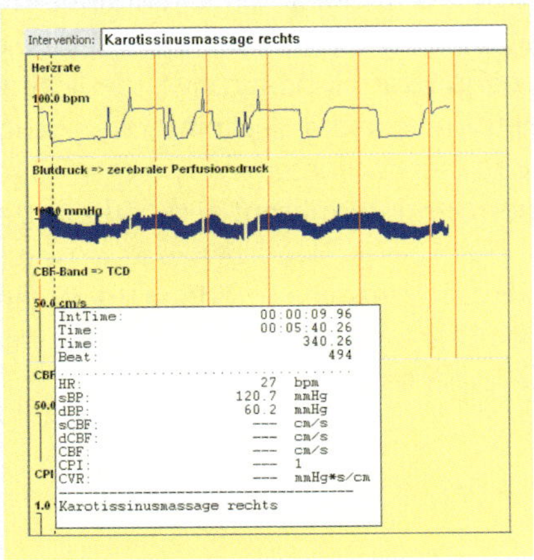

Figure 40 Bradycardia and subsequently occurring fall in blood pressure during carotid sinus massage.

The patient's medical history and documented hemodynamic parameters during carotid sinus massage led to the conclusion that dual chamber pacing is indicated.

4 Appendix

4.1 Model of a diagnostically relevant patient questionnaire for syncope diagnosis

Medical history taking is a crucial tool for the diagnosis and differential diagnosis of syncope. In some cases the medical history alone can lead to a diagnosis, e.g., a diagnosis of vasovagal syncope after prolonged standing, in "stuffy air" and with typical prodromal symptoms (sensation of physical alienation, vertigo, nausea, pallor), in other situations it provides a means of guiding the subsequent diagnostic strategy. Incomplete medical histories can lead to medical examinations that are stressful for patients, possibly obstruct the actual diagnosis and are economically inefficient.

The first question to consider is whether the symptoms correspond to the definition of syncope or if the symptoms only resemble syncopal attacks. The next step involves differentiating the underlying possible causes.

The model described below consists of two parts: In part 1, patients are informed about the suspected diagnosis and in part 2, the purpose of the questionnaire is outlined.

For other information sheets (some also with illustrations) including consent forms, see the website www.synkope.at.

4.1.1 Information sheet

Information for patients referred with a suspected diagnosis of "syncope"

Dear Sir or Madam,

You have been admitted to our hospital because of suspected transient loss of consciousness. A short, transient loss of consciousness that ends spontaneously and is followed by complete recovery, usually associated with a loss of voluntary muscle tone and falling, is medically referred to as "syncope".
The assessment of syncope is of considerable importance, first, because it may be a manifestation of a possibly serious underlying disorder, and second, because it entails a high risk of injury due to accidents and falls. The attached questionnaire represents a tool which helps us to determine the cause of your syncopal events. Answering these questions will help us to obtain an accurate and complete impression of your symptoms and to initiate any necessary diagnostic and treatment strategies. This questionnaire is not supposed to replace a personal audience with the attending physician, but rather to complete it.
Please take your time to answer the questions. Sometimes it may be important to question people who have witnessed your symptoms to obtain necessary information about the exact circumstances.
If you have any questions, please don't hesitate to ask staff on your ward. They will be happy to help, and your information and answers will be treated confidentially.

With best wishes for your recovery,

Your hospital team

4.1.2 Patient questionnaire

Questionnaire

1. Have your symptoms ever been followed by a short loss of consciousness?	☐ yes	☐ no
2. If yes, how many seconds were you unconscious?		seconds
3. Did your muscle tone get weak, did you "slump over"?	☐ yes	☐ no
4. Have you ever had an associated injury that needed medical attention?	☐ yes	☐ no
If yes, what kind of injury?		
Kind of injury:		
5. Did you feel anxiety or pain, or did you sense a very disagreeable smell or an unpleasant noise before the loss of consciousness occurred?	☐ yes	☐ no
6. Did your loss of consciousness occur after prolonged standing (> 5 minutes)?	☐ yes	☐ no
7. Did your loss of consciousness occur immediately after a considerable exertion and are you free of any cardiac diseases?	☐ yes	☐ no
8. Did your loss of consciousness occur during a considerable exertion and do you suffer of any cardiac disease (no matter which kind of cardiac disease)?	☐ yes	☐ no
9. Do you have a family history of death associated with unexplained loss of consciousness or with sudden cardiac death?	☐ yes	☐ no
10. Was your loss of consciousness very short and without any premonitory symptoms, and do you have a cardiac disease or a cardiac pacemaker?	☐ yes	☐ no
11. Did you experience palpitations or irregular heartbeats before the loss of consciousness?	☐ yes	☐ no
12. Did you experience severe difficulties in breathing or chest pain before the loss of consciousness?	☐ yes	☐ no
13. Did the loss of consciousness occur immediately after urination, coughing, swallowing or after bowel movements?	☐ yes	☐ no

14. Did the loss of consciousness occur within a few seconds after standing up from a lying position?	☐ yes	☐ no
15. Did the loss of consciousness occur after lying down after sitting or after turning around when you were already lying?	☐ yes	☐ no
16. Did the loss of consciousness occur after sudden head rotation or after pressure on the neck, e.g., during shaving, by tight collars or after shouldering a heavy load?	☐ yes	☐ no
17. If you are on medication: Has the dosage been changed recently?	☐ yes	☐ no
18. Was the loss of consciousness accompanied by one of the following symptoms: tongue biting, twitching movements or bluish face?	☐ yes	☐ no
19. Were you confused for more than 5 minutes and not "quite yourself" after regaining consciousness?	☐ yes	☐ no
20. Did you smell or taste anything unusual before the loss of consciousness occurred?	☐ yes	☐ no
21. Did the loss of consciousness occur after vigorous exercise of one or both arms?	☐ yes	☐ no
22. Did the loss of consciousness occur in the middle of a crush or in a crowded place?	☐ yes	☐ no
23. Do the symptoms occur often (> once per month), and have you sought clinical advice but without any result as to the cause of the attacks?	☐ yes	☐ no
24. Was the loss of consciousness preceded mostly by vertigo?	☐ yes	☐ no
25. Was the loss of consciousness accompanied by speech disorders or double vision?	☐ yes	☐ no
26. Was the loss of consciousness accompanied by intense facial pain?	☐ yes	☐ no
27. Did the loss of consciousness occur ~1 hour after a meal?	☐ yes	☐ no
28. Was the loss of consciousness accompanied by violent headaches?	☐ yes	☐ no

4.2 Differential diagnosis and diagnostic algorithm

The questions in part 2 of the questionnaire are assigned to specific subject complexes in a systematic way and serve as a guiding tool for the attendant physician. The answers to these questions are intended to complement the medical history taken by the physician because it is impossible to ask all features that are clinically relevant for syncope and for clinical manifestations resembling syncope during a patient-doctor-conversation.

The chosen questions provide indications of typical circumstances, without being diagnostic by themselves or showing a clear-cut definable specificity or sensitivity. They represent, however, the current school of thought and the essence of what is generally considered as "typical". If the analysis of the questionnaire emphasizes one category, then this is the one that diagnostic measures – if still considered necessary – should first focus on.

Part 3 describes the connection of the questions to defined clinical manifestations. Part 4 describes the example of a decision algorithm – derived on the basis of this questionnaire – that is already in use.

In view of the development of "disease management programs" and in consideration of resources becoming scarcer, the implementation of an algorithm-oriented clinical pathway seems to be urgently called for.

4.2.1 Correspondence of question complexes

Table 15 Correspondence of question complexes to possibly underlying disorder

Question number	Etiology/medical history pointing towards
1–4	Differentiation: syncope or non-syncopal condition?
5–7	Vasovagal syncope
8–12	Syncope associated with structural heart and/or cardiopulmonary disease (e.g. valvular heart disease, pulmonary hypertension, pulmonary embolism, hypertrophic (obstructive) cardiomyopathy, arrhythmias including brady- or tachycardias, etc.)
13	Situational syncope
14	Orthostatic hypotension
15	Atrial thrombus/myxoma
16	Carotid sinus hypersensitivity
17	Drug-induced syncope
18–20	Epilepsy
21	Subclavian steal syndrome
22–23	Psychiatric disorder
24–25	TIA in the vertebrobasilar circulation
26	Trigeminal/glossopharyngeal neuralgia
27	Dumping syndrome or post-prandial due to autonomic failure
28	Migraine

4.2.2 Diagnostic algorithm

Diagnostic pathway for the assessment of syncopal attacks

If medical history reveals presence of syncope according to the definition: *"transient self-limited loss of consciousness with sudden loss of voluntary muscle tone"*, then follow:

I. Routine evaluations

1. *Medical history* (including current medication, previous diseases and co-morbidities, among others: epilepsy/structural heart disease/pulmonary disease/thromboses and embolisms/cerebral apoplexy/psychiatric disorder/migraine/family history, particularly regarding similar symptoms or sudden cardiac death, Parkinson's disease, narcolepsy, diabetes mellitus, questions about previous surgery, especially of the digestive system)

2. *Syncope questionnaire*

3. *Physical examination* (especially cardiac murmur when supine and during change of posture, inflow congestion, cyanosis, tongue bite, signs of dehydration, signs of blood loss, pallor, paresis, trigeminal trigger points, pulse state, etc.)

4. *Blood pressure monitoring after RR in both arms*

5. *12-lead ECG*

6. *Measurement of blood glucose*

If routine evaluation findings already point towards a possible etiology, then it should be followed by individual diagnostic evaluation, e.g. in the case of suspected valvular heart disease immediate echocardiography, in the case of blood pressure differences in both arms immediate duplex ultrasonography of the subclavian artery, in the case of suspected acute coronary ischemia its immediate exclusion or acute coronary angiography, etc.
Syncope questionnaire analysis: If there is one "yes" in the boxes of 5–7, or 8–12, or 13, or 14, or 15, or 16, or 17, or 18–20, or 21, or 22–23, or 24–25, or 26, or 27, or 28, then the analysis should be followed by **basic evaluation** of each complex, starting with the potentially most dangerous disorder.

If the subsequent diagnostic measures yield a certain diagnosis, there is no need for further diagnostic evaluations. In absence of a diagnostic result, the patient is to be re-evaluated, followed by individual diagnostic measures or no further diagnostic measures, if:

a) Probable benign character of syncope[1, 4] (no high-risk occupation (pilot, bus operator, physician), rare occurrence (not more often than once per year), age < 35 years, absence of structural heart disease, no serious injuries)
b) Probability of vasovagal syncope[5]
c) Orthostatic hypotension

II. Diagnostic pathway following the questionnaire

Questions 5–7 (vasovagal syncope)
Basic evaluation: tilt table testing (as described in [1])

Questions 8–12 (associated with structural heart and/or cardiopulmonary disease)
Basic evaluation:
1. Exclusion of acute coronary ischemia (laboratory tests: biomarkers at intervals of 3 hours + repeated ECG 3 hours after ECG upon admission)
2. Echocardiography

Further diagnostic measures depending upon the results of step 1 (ECG) and 2 (Echo). If there is no evidence of acute coronary ischemia then an exercise test should follow.

In the following cases echocardiography is diagnostic and the underlying disease requires further diagnostic measures, e.g.:

Dilated CMP, low LV-EF	Holter monitoring with HR-variability, coronary angiography, and, if necessary, EPS
HOCM	Gradient assessment, and, if necessary, provocation test, Holter monitoring with HR-variability, medical history, family history of sudden cardiac death (SCD)
Right ventricular strain	Exclusion of pulmonary embolus (scintillation scanning or CT), capillary or arterial ABG, right heart catheterization, chest radiography
Myxoma, NPL, Thrombus	Transesophageal echocardiography (TEE), MRT

Valvular heart disease	TEE and invasive assessment (right and left heart catheterization)
Aortic dissection	TEE, computer tomography
Pericardial effusion	If necessary, pericardial drainage for diagnostic (and therapeutic) purpose. Further diagnostic procedures according to the suspected underlying disease
Right ventricular dysplasia	Medical history, family history of sudden cardiac death, Holter monitoring with HR-variability, MRT, consider EPS

If there is evidence of acute coronary ischemia, then immediate coronary angiography/PCI should follow.
If routine ECG is abnormal but without evidence of acute coronary ischemia, then further diagnostic steps, depending upon the concrete ECG, are recommended, e.g.:

Prolonged, not drug-induced QT-interval	Medical history, family history, consider EPS
Brugada syndrome	Medical history, family history, consider EPS
Bradycardia (not drug-induced)	Holter monitoring, consider pacemaker implantation
Tachycardia (not drug-induced)	Holter monitoring, consider pharmacologic treatment or ICD

If the previous diagnostic measures do not yield any diagnosis, then Holter monitoring should follow. If this work-up is not diagnostic, a prolonged monitoring strategy is recommended with external or implantable event-recorders.

Question 13 (situational syncope)
Basic evaluation: No further diagnostic procedures recommended

Question 14 (orthostatic hypotension)
Basic evaluation: Schellong test (as described in [6])

Question 15 (atrial thrombus/myxoma [or another kind of tumor])
Basic evaluation: Transthoracic and transesophageal echocardiography, MRT

Question 16 (carotid sinus hypersensitivity)
Basic evaluation: Carotid sinus massage (as described in [7, 8])

Question 17 (medication related)
Basic evaluation: Evaluation and, if necessary, modification of medication, preferring agents with prolonged half-time and one-time administration

Questions 18–20 (indication of epilepsy)
Basic evaluation: Consultation of a neurologist, and further procedures depending upon the result, most likely CCT and EEG

Question 21 (indication of subclavian steal syndrome)
Basic evaluation: Duplex ultrasonography

Questions 22–23 (indication of psychiatric disorder)
Basic evaluation: Consultation of a psychiatrist, and further procedures depending upon the results

Questions 24–25 (indication of TIA in the vertebrobasilar circulation)
Basic evaluation: Duplex ultrasonography of extracranial brain-supplying arteries, and, if warranted by resulting findings, CCT and transcranial duplex ultrasonography

Question 26 (indication of trigeminal/glossopharyngeal neuralgia)
Basic evaluation: Consultation of a neurologist, and further procedures depending upon the results

Question 27 (post-prandial or dumping syndrome)
Basic evaluation: No further diagnostic procedures recommended

Question 28 (migraine)
Basic evaluation: Consultation of a neurologist, and further procedures depending upon the results

Sources:

[1] Task Force of The European Society of Cardiology and The North American Society of Pacing and Electrophysiology. Heart rate variability: Standards of measurement, physiological interpretation, and clinical use. Eur Heart J 1996; 17: 354–381.
[2] Kapoor WN. Syncope. New Engl J Med 2000; 343(25):1856–1862.
[3] Kardiologie Campus Virchow-Klinikum & Campus Berlin-Buch. Synkopenabklärung. Leitlinienbasierte Therapieempfehlungen. Kardiologie CVK & CBB 1–4 (2002).
[4] Marti B, Villiger B, Hintermann M, Lerch R. Plötzlicher Herztod beim Sport: Sinnvolle Vorsorgeuntersuchungen und Präventionsmassnahmen.

Schweizerische Zeitschrift für "Sportmedizin und Sporttraumatologie" 1998; 46(2): 83–85.
[5] Kapoor WN, Smith M, Miller NL. Upright tilt testing in evaluating syncope: a comprehensive literature review. Am J Med 1994; 97: 78–88.
[6] The Consensus Committee of the American Autonomic Society and the American Academy of Neurology. Consensus statement on the definition of orthostatic hypotension, pure autonomic failure, and multiple system atrophy. Neurology 1996; 46: 1470.
[7] Brignole M, Sartore B, Prato R. Role of body position during carotid sinus stimulation test in the diagnosis of cardioinhibitory carotid sinus syndrome. G Ital Cardiol 1983; 14: 69–72.
[8] Parry SW, Richardson D, O'Shea D, Sen B, Kenny RA. Diagnosis of carotid sinus hypersensitivity in older adults: Carotid sinus massage in the upright position is essential. Heart 2000; 83: 22–23.

4.3 Normal values[1]

1. Hemodynamic parameters

Parameter	Abbrevation	Unit	Normal value
Heart rate	HR	bpm	60–90
RR-Interval	RRI	ms	660–1000
Systolic blood pressure	sBP	mmHg	90–129
Diastolic blood pressure	dBP	mmHg	50–84
Mean arterial blood pressure	mBP	mmHg	< 100
Stroke volume	SV	ml	60–120
Stroke index	SI	ml/m^2	30–80
Cardiac output	CO	L/min	4–8
Cardiac index	CI	$L/min/m^2$	2.5–4.5
Total peripheral resistance	TPR	$dyn*s/cm^5$	900–1200
Acceleration index	ACI	$100/s^2$	50–150
Index of contractility	IC	1000/s	33–65
Maximum rise in pressure	dP/dt_{max}	mmHg/s	500–1000

1 [72,148,174,307,335].

2. Cardiovascular autonomic function: Baroreflex sensitivity[2]

Age-related normal value	**Baroreflex sensitivity: Slope**	**Baroreflex sensitivity: Event-count/10 min**
18–29 years		
Men	14.0	26.2
Women	13.7	28.7
30–39 years		
Men	10.6	18.8
Women	9.9	19.3
40–49 years		
Men	8.1	19.7
Women	7.6	18.8
50–60 years		
Men	6.0	17.3
Women	7.3	16.9

3. Cardiovascular autonomic function: Heart rate variability[3]

Heart rate variability LF (0.04–0.15 Hz)	LF_RRI	ms^2	1170 ± 416
Heart rate variability HF (0.15–0.4 Hz)	HF_RRI	ms^2	975 ± 203
Normalized units LF	LFnu_RRI	%	54 ± 4
Normalized units HF	HFnu_RRI	%	29 ± 3
Power spectral density	PSD_RRI	ms^2	3466 ± 1018
Sympatho-vagal balance (LF_RRI/HF_RRI)	LF/HF	–	1.5–2

2 [148] Normal values of these parameters are, among others, particularly age- and sex-related (see Chapter 1.5.1).

3 [307] Normal values are subject to variations, depending upon the chosen measuring method; the values mentioned here are related to a measuring period of 5 minutes with the patient lying supine (see Chapter 1.5.1). They are not validated to be used as a basis for clinical decision processes.

5 Bibliography

A thematically structured bibliography is available on the internet (www.synkope.at).

[1] Aaronson KD, Schwartz JS, Chen TM, et al. Development and prospective validation of a clinical index to predict survival in ambulatory patients referred for cardiac transplant evaluation. Circulation 1997;95:2660–2667.

[2] Abe H, Kondo S, Koshi K, et al. Usefulness of orthostatic self-training for the prevention of neurocardiogenic syncope. Pacing Clin Electrophysiol 2002;25:1454–1458.

[3] Abi-Samra F, Maloney JD, Fouad-Tarazi FM, Castle L. The usefulness of head-up tilt testing and hemodynamic investigations in the workup of syncope of unknown origin. PACE 1988;11:1202–1214.

[4] Abraham WT, Fisher WG, Smith AL, Delurgio DB, Leon AR, Loh E, Kocovic DZ, Packer M, Clavell AL, Hayes DL, Ellestad M, Trupp RJ, Underwood J, Pickering F, Truex C, McAtee P, Messenger J; MIRACLE Study Group. Multicenter InSync Randomized Clinical Evaluation. Cardiac resynchronization in chronic heart failure. N Engl J Med 2002;346:1845–1853.

[5] Adamson PB, Huang MH, Vanoli E, Foreman RD, Schwartz PJ, Hull SS Jr. Unexpected interaction between β-adrenergic blockade and heart rate variability before and after myocardial infarction: a longitudinal study in dogs at high and low risk for sudden death. Circulation 1994;90:976–982.

[6] Akselrod S, Gordon D, Ubel FA, Shannon DC, Barger AC, Cohen RJ. Power spectrum analysis of heart rate fluctuation: a quantitative probe of beat to beat cardiovascular control. Science 1981;213:220–222.

[7] Albina G, Fernandez Cisneros L, Laino R, Nobo UL, Ortega D, Schwarz E, Barja L, Lagos R, Giniger A, Ameriso SF. Transcranial Doppler monitoring during head upright tilt table testing in patients with suspected neurocardiogenic syncope. Europace 2004;6:63–69.

[8] Allen SC, Taylor CL, Hall VE. A study of orthostatic insufficiency by the tiltboard method. Am J Physiol 1945;143:11.
[9] Almquist A, Goldenberg IF, Milstein S, et al. Provocation of bradycardia and hypotension by isoproterenol and upright posture in patients with unexplained syncope. N Engl J Med 1989;320:346–351.
[10] Anguita M, Arizon J, Bueno G, Latre J, Sancho M, Torres F, Gimenez D, Concha M, Valles F. Clinical and hemodynamic predictors of survival in patients aged <65 years with severe congestive heart failure secondary to ischemic or nonischemic dilated cardiomyopathy. Am J Cardiol 1993;72: 413–417.
[11] Atzler E, Lehmann D. Über ein neues Verfahren zur Darstellung der Herztätigkeit (Dielektrographie). Arbeitsphysiologie 1932;6:636–680.
[12] Auricchio A, Stellbrink C, Block M, et al. Effect of pacing chamber and atrioventricular delay on acute systolic function of paced patients with congestive heart failure. Circulation 1999;99:2993–3001.
[13] Bannister R, Mathias C. Introduction and classification of autonomic disorders. In: Mathias CJ, Bannister R, eds. Autonomic failure, 4th edn. Oxford: Oxford University Press 1999:xvii–xxii.
[14] Bartoletti A, Gaggioli G, Bottoni N et al. Head-up tilt testing potentiated with oral nitroglycerin. A randomized trial of the contribution of a drug-free phase and a nitroglycerin phase in the diagnosis of neurally mediated syncope. Europace 1999;1:83–86.
[15] Benditt DG, Brignole M. Syncope: Is a diagnosis a diagnosis? JACC 2003;41(5):791–794.
[16] Benditt DG, Ferguson DW, Grubb BP, et al. Tilt-table testing for assessing syncope. An American College of Cardiology expert consensus document. J Am Coll Cardiol 1996;28:263–275.
[17] Benditt DG, Remole S, Bailin S, Dunnigan A, Asso A, Milstein S. Tilt table testing for evaluation of neurally-mediated (cardioneurogenic) syncope: rationale and proposed protocols. PACE 1991;14:1528–1537.
[18] Benditt DG, Sakaguchi S, JJ, Remole S, Adler S, Lurie KG. Syncope. Diagnostic considerations and the role of tilt table testing. Cardiol Rev 1993;1:146 –156.
[19] Benditt DG. Cardiac pacing for prevention of vasovagal syncope (editorial). J Am Coll Cardiol 1999;33:21–23.
[20] Bernstein DP. A new stroke volume equation for thoracic electrical bioimpedance: theory and rationale. Crit Care Med 1986;14(10):904–909.
[21] Bernstein DP. Continuous noninvasive real-time monitoring of stroke volume and cardiac output by thoracic electrical bioimpedance. Crit Care Med 1986;14(10):898–901.

[22] Bertinieri G, Di Renzo M, Cavallazi A. A new approach to analysis of the arterial baroreflex. J Hypertens Suppl. 1985;3(3):79–81.
[23] Betz R, Bastanier CK, Mocellin R. Die Impedanzkardiographie als Methode zur quantitativen Bestimmung des Herzzeitvolumens. Vergleichende Messungen mit dem Fickschen Prinzip. Basic Res. Cardiol. 1977;72: 46–56.
[24] Biffi M, Boriani G, Sabbatani P, et al. Malignant vasovagal syncope: a randomised trial of metoprolol and clonidine. Heart 1997;77:268–272.
[25] Bigger JT Jr, Fleiss JL, Steimnan RC, Rolnitzky LM, Kleiger RE, Rottman JN. Frequency domain measures of heart period variability and mortality after myocardial infarction. Circulation 1992;85:164–171.
[26] Bigger JT, Fleiss JL, Rolnitzky LM, Steinman RC. The ability of several short-term measures of RR variability to predict mortality after myocardial infarction. Circulation 1993;88:927–934.
[27] Billman GE, Schwartz PJ, Stone HL. Baroreceptor reflex control of heart rate: a predictor of sudden cardiac death. Circulation 1982;66:874–880.
[28] Billman GE, Schwartz PJ, Stone HL. The effects of daily exercise on susceptibility to sudden cardiac death. Circulation 1984;69:1182–1189.
[29] Blanc JJ, Genet L, Mansourati J, et al. Interêt du test d'inclinaison dans le diagnostic etiologique des pertes de connaissance. Presse Med 1990;19: 857–859.
[30] Blanc JJ, Mansourati J, Maheu B, Boughaleb D, Genet L. Reproducibility of a positive passive upright tilt test at a seven-day interval in patients with syncope. Am J Cardiol 1993;72:469–471.
[31] Braune S, Lücking CH. Orthostatische Hypotonie: Pathophysiologie, Differentialdiagnose und Therapie. Deutsches Ärzteblatt 1997;50:A-3413.
[32] Brembilla-Perrot B, Suty-Selton C, Houriez P, Claudon O, Beurrier D, de la Chaise AT. Value of non-invasive and invasive studies in patients with bundle branch block, syncope and history of myocardial infarction, Europace 2001;3(3):187–194.
[33] Brignole M, Alboni P, Benditt D, Bergfeldt L, Blanc JJ, Bloch Thomsen PE, van Dijk JG, Fitzpatrick A, Hohnloser S, Janousek J, Kapoor W, Kenny RA, Kulakowski P, Moya A, Raviele A, Sutton R, Theodorakis G, Wieling W. Task Force Report: Guidelines on management (diagnosis and treatment) of syncope. Eur Heart J 2001;22 1256–1306.
[34] Brignole M, Alboni P, Benditt D, Bergfeldt L, Blanc JJ, Bloch Thomsen PE, van Dijk JG, Fitzpatrick A, Hohnloser S, Janousek J, Kapoor W, Kenny RA, Kulakowski P, Masotti G, Moya A, Raviele A, Sutton R, Theodorakis G, Ungar A, Wieling W. Guidelines on management (diagnosis and treatment) of syncope – Update 2004 Eur Heart J 2004;25:2054–2072.

[35] Brignole M, Croci F, Menozzi C, et al. Isometric arm counter-pressure maneuvers to abort impending vasovagal syncope. J Am Coll Cardiol 2002;40:2054–2060.
[36] Brignole M, Menozzi C, Del Rosso A, et al. New classiflcation of haemodynamics of vasovagal syncope: beyond the VASIS classification. Analysis of the pre-syncopal phase of the tilt test without and with nitroglycerin challenge. Europace 2000;2:66–76.
[37] Brignole M, Menozzi C, Gianfranchi L, Oddone D, Lolli G, Bertulla A. Carotid sinus massage, eyeball compression and head-up tilt test in patients with syncope of uncertain origin and in healthy control subjects. Am Heart J 1991;122:1644–1651.
[38] Brignole M, Menozzi C, Gianfranci L, et al. Neurally mediated syncope detected by carotid sinus massage and head up tilt in sick sinus syndrome. Am J Cardiol 1991;68:1032–1036.
[39] Brignole M, Menozzi C, Gianfranci L, Lolli G, Bottoni N, Oddone D. A controlled trial of acute and long-term medical therapy in tilt-induced neurally mediated syncope. Am J Cardiol 1992;70:339–342.
[40] Brignole M, Menozzi C, Lolli G, Bottoni N, Gaggioli G. Long-term outcome of paced and non paced patients with severe carotid sinus syndrome. Am J Cardiol 1992;69:1039–1043.
[41] Brignole M, Menozzi C, Lolli G, Oddone D, Gianfranchi L, Bertulla A. Validation of a method for choice of pacing mode in carotid sinus syndrome with or without sinus bradycardia. PACE 1991;14:196–203.
[42] Brignole M, Sartore B, Prato R. Role of body position during carotid sinus stimulation test in the diagnosis of cardioinhibitory carotid sinus syndrome. G Ital Cardiol 1983;14:69–72.
[43] Brignole M, Sartore B. Barra M. Menozzi C. Lolli G. Ventricular and dual chamber pacing for treatment of carotid sinus syndrome. PACE 1989;12: 582–590.
[44] Brignole M. Sartore B, Barra M. Menozzi C, Lolli G. Is DDD superonr to VVI pacing in mixed carotid sinus syndrome? An acute and medium-term study. PACE 1988;11:1902–1910.
[45] Bristow MR, Feldman AM, Saxon LA. Heart failure management using implantable devices for ventricular resynchronization: Comparison of medical therapy, pacing, and defibrillation in chronic heart failure (COMPANION) trial. COMPANION Steering Committee and COMPANION Clinical Investigators. J Card Fail 2000;6(3):276–85.
[46] Brooks R, Ruskin JN, Powell AC, Newell J, Garan H, Mcgovern BA. Prospective evaluation of day-to-day reproducibility of upright tilt table testing in unexplained syncope. Am J Cardiol 1993;71:1289–1292.

[47] Brown AM, Malliani A. Spinal sympathetic reflexes initiated by coronary receptors. J Physiol 1971;212:685–705.

[48] Brown AP, Dawkins KD, Davies JG. Detection of arrhythmias: use of a patient-activated ambulatory electrocardiogram device with a solid-state memory loop. Br Heart J 1987;58:251–253.

[49] Calkins H, Byrne M, El-Atassi R, Kalbfleisch S, Langberg JL, Morady F. The economic burden of unrecognised vasodepressor syncope. Am J Med 1993;95:473–479.

[50] Campana C, Gavazzi A, Berzuini C, Larizza C, Marioni R, D'Armini A, Pederzolli N, Martinelli L, Vigano M. Predictors of prognosis in patients awaiting heart transplantation. J Heart Lung Transplant 1993;12:756–765.

[51] Campbell A, Reinken J, Allen B, et al. Falls in old age: A study of frequency and related clinical factors. Age and Ageing 1981;10:264–270.

[52] Carey BJ, Eames PJ, Panerai RB, et al. Carbon dioxide, critical closing pressure and cerebral haemodynamics prior to vasovagal syncope in humans. Clin Sci 2001;101:351–358.

[53] Casolo GC, Stroder P, Signorini C, Calzolari F, Zucchini M, Balli E, Sulla A, Lazzerini S. Heart rate variability during the acute phase of myocardial infarction. Circulation 1992;85:2073–2079.

[54] Charité Berlin: Leitlinienbasierte Therapieempfehlung zur Synkopenabklärung 2002. www.fvk-berlin.de/fvkweb/fvkindex.html.

[55] Chen XC, Chen MY, Remole S, et al. Reproducibility of head up tilt table testing for eliciting susceptibility to neurally-mediated syncope in patients without structural heart disease. Am J Cardiol 1992;69:755–760.

[56] Christensen JH, Gustenhoff P, Korup E, Aaroe J, Toft E, Moller J, Rasmussen K, Dyerberg J, Schmidt EB. Effect of fish oil on heart rate variability in survivors of myocardial infarction: a double blind randomised controlled trial. BMJ 1996;312:677–678.

[57] Christensen JH, Skou HA, Fog L, Hansen V, Vesterlund T, Dyerberg J, Toft E, Schmidt EB. Marine n-3 fatty acids, wine intake, and heart rate variability in patients referred for coronary angiography. Circulation 2001;103:651–657.

[58] Cohen MB, Snow JS, Grasso V, et al. Efficacy of pindolol for treatment of vasovagal syncope. Am Heart J 1995;130:786–790.

[59] Cohn J, Johnson G, Shabetai R, Loeb H, Tristani F, Rector T, Smith R, Fletcher R, for the V-HeFT VA Cooperative Studies Group. Ejection fraction, peak exercise oxygen consumption, cardiothoracic ratio, ventricular arrhythmias, and plasma norepinephrine as determinants of prognosis in heart failure. Circulation 1993;87(suppl VI):VI-5–VI-16.

[60] Cohn J, Levine T, Olivari M, Garberg V, Lura D, Francis G, Simon A, Rector T. Plasma norepinephrine as a guide to prognosis in patients with chronic congestive heart failure. N Engl J Med 1984;311:819–823.

[61] Cohn J, Rector T. Prognosis of congestive heart failure and predictors of mortality. Am J Cardiol 1988;62:25A–30A.

[62] Connolly SJ, Sheldon R, Roberts RS, Gent M. The North American Vasovagal Pacemaker Study (VPS). A randomized trial of permanent cardiac pacing for the prevention of vasovagal syncope. J Am Coll Cardiol. 1999;33(1):16–20.

[63] Connolly SJ, Sheldon R, Thorpe KE, Roberts RS, Ellenbogen KA, Wilkoff BL, Morillo C, Gent M; VPS II Investigators. Pacemaker therapy for prevention of syncope in patients with recurrent severe vasovagal syncope: Second Vasovagal Pacemaker Study (VPS II): a randomized trial. JAMA 2003;289(17):2224–2229.

[64] Consensus Committee of the American Autonomic Society and the American Academy of Neurology. Consensus statement on the definition of orthostatic hypotension, pure autonomic failure, and multiple system atrophy. J Neurol Sci 1996;144:218–219.

[65] Corr PB, Yamada KA, Witkowski FX. Mechanisms controlling cardiac autonomic function and their relation to arrhythmogenesis. In: Fozzard HA, Haber E, Jennings RB, Katz AN, Morgan HE, eds. The Heart and Cardiovascular System. New York, NY: Raven Press 1986:1343–1403.

[66] Cottier C. Kurzdauernde Bewusstlosigkeit (Synkopen) Teil 1: Einführung und Abklärungsgang bei Synkopen. PRAXIS Schweiz Med Forum 2002;18:430–436.

[67] Credner SC, Klingenheben T. Kardiogene Synkopen: Ursachen und differentialdiagnostisches Vorgehen. herzmedizin 2002;19(4):195–199.

[68] Cummings SR, Rubin SM, Black D. The future of hip fractures in the United States. Numbers, costs, and potential effects of postmenopausal estrogen. Clin Orthopaedics and Related Res 1990;252:163–166.

[69] Dalal P, Fujisic K, Hupart P, Schwietzer P. Arrhythmogenic right ventricular dysplasia: a review. Cardiology 1994;85:361–369.

[70] Dalla Pozza R, Kleinmann A, Zysk S, Bechtold S, Netz N. Head-up-tilt testing in children: new perspectives using beat-to-beat blood-pressure monitoring. Images Pediatr Cardiol 2005;22:1–7.

[71] Davies AJ, Kenny RA. Incidence of complications after carotid sinus massage in older patients with syncope. Am J Cardiol 1998;81:1256–1257.

[72] Dawson SL, Robinson TG, Youhde JH, James MA, Martin A, Weston P, Paneral R, Potter JF. The reproducibility of cardiac baroreceptor activity assessed non-invasively by spectral and sequence techniques. Clin Auton Res 1997;7:279–284.

[73] Day SC, Cook EF, Funkenstein H, Goldman L. Evaluation and outcome of emergency room patients with transient loss of consciousness. Am J Med 1982;73:15–23.

[74] De Mey C, Enterling D. Variant responses impair the usefulness of passive upright tilt in drug research. Methods Find Exp Clin Pharmacol 1988;10: 57–64.

[75] Del Rosso A, Bartoletti A, Bartoli P, Ungar A, Bonechi F, Maioli M, Ieri A. Methodology of head-up tilt testing potentiated with sublingual nitrogycerin in unexplained syncope, Am J Cardiol 2000;85:1007–1001.

[76] Deschamps D, Richard A, Citron D, Chaperon A. Biaon JP. Ponsonaille J. Hypersensibilite sino-carotidienne. Evolution à moyen et à long tertne des patients traités par stimulation ventriculaire. Arch Mal Coeur 1990;83: 63–67.

[77] Deutsche Gesellschaft für Kardiologie – Herz- und Kreislaufforschung Richtlinien für die Durchführung der nicht-invasiven Diagnostik von Rhythmusstörungen, Z Kardiol 1999;88:51–60.

[78] Di Girolamo E, Di Iorio C, Leonzio L, Sabatini P, Barsotti A. Usefulness of a tilt training program for the prevention of refractory neurocardiogenic syncope in adolescents. A controlled study. Circulation 1999;100:1798–1801.

[79] Di Girolamo E, Di Iorio C, Sabatini O. Leonzio L. Barbone C, Barsotti A. Effects of paroxetine hydrochloride, a selective serotonin reuptake inhibitor, on refractory vasovagal syncope: a randomized, double-blind, placebo-controlled study. J Am Coll Cardiol 1999;33:1227–1230.

[80] Diehl, RR. Posturales Tachykardiesyndrom: In Deutschland bislang zu selten diagnostiziert. Deutsches Ärzteblatt 2003;43:A–2794.

[81] Dietary supplementation with n-3 polyunsaturated fatty acids and vitamin E after myocardial infarction: results of the GISSI-Prevenzione trial. Gruppo Italiano per lo Studio della Sopravvivenza nell'Infarto miocardico. Lancet 1999;354:447–455.

[82] Eagle KA, Black HR, Cook EF. Evaluation of prognostic classification for patients with syncope. Am J Med 1985;79:455–460.

[83] Ector H, Reybrouck T, Heidbuchel H, Gewillig M, Van de Werf F. Tilt training: a new treatment for recurrent neurocardiogenic syncope or severe orthostatic intolerance. PACE 1998;21:193–196.

[84] El-Bedawi KM. Wahbha MMMAE, Hainsworth R. Cardiac pacing does not improvce orthostatic tolerance in patients with vasovagal syncope. Clin Autonom Res 1995;88:463–470.

[85] Ewing DJ, Martin CN, Young RJ, Clarke BF. The value of cardiovascular autonomic function tests: 10 years' experience in diabetes. Diabetes Care 1985;8:491–498.

[86] Farrell TG, Bashir Y, Cripps T, et al. Risk stratification for arrhythmic events in postinfarction patients based on heart rate variability, ambulatory electrocardiographic variables and the signal-averaged electrocardiogram. J Am Coll Cardiol 1991;18:687–697.

[87] Farrell TG, Odemuyiwa O, Bashir Y, Cripps TR, Malik M, Ward DE, Camm AJ. Prognostic value of baroreflex sensitivity testing after acute myocardial infarction. Br Heart J 1992;67:129–137.

[88] Fish FA, Strasburger JF, Benson DW. Reproducibility of a symptomatic response to upright tilt in young patients with unexplained syncope. Am J Cardiol 1992;70:605–609.

[89] Fitzpatrick A, Sutton R. Tilting towards a diagnosis in unexplained syncope. Lancet 1989;1:658–660.

[90] Fitzpatrick A, Theodorakis G, Vardas P, Sutton R. Methodology of head-up tilt testing in patients with unexplained syncope. J Am Coll Cardiol 1991;17:125–130.

[91] Fitzpatrick A. Theodorakis G. Ahmed R, Williams T. Sutton R. Dual chamber pacing aborts vasovagal syncope induced by head-up 60 degree tilt. PACE 1991;14;13–19.

[92] Fitzpatrick AP, Ahmed R, Williams S, et al. A randomized trial of medical therapy in malignant vasovagal syndrome or neurally-mediated bradycardia/hypotension syndrome. Eur J Cardiac Pacing Electrophysiol 1991;1: 191–202.

[93] Flevari PP, Livanis EG, Theodorakis GN, Mesiskli T, Zarvalis E, Kremastinos DT. Baroreflexes in vasovagal syncope: Two types of abnormal response. J of Pacing Clin Electrophysiol 2002;25(9):1315–1323.

[94] Foglia Manzillo G, Giada F, Bcretta S, Corrado G, Santarone M, Raviele A. Reproducibility of head-up tilt testing potentiated with sublingual nitroglycerin in patients with unexplained syncope. Am J Cardiol 1999;84:284–288.

[95] Fortin J, Habenbacher W, Heller A, Hacker A, Grüllenberger R, Innerhofer J, Passath H, Wagner Ch, Haitchi G, Flotzinger D, Pacher R, Wach P. Non-invasive beat-to-beat cardiac output monitoring by an improved method of transthoracic bioimpedance measurement. Comp Biol Med 2005: accepted for publication.

[96] Fortin J, Marte W, Grüllenberger R, Hacker A, Habenbacher W, Heller A, Wagner Ch, Wach P, Skrabal F. Continuous non-invasive blood pressure monitoring using concentrically interlocking control loops. Comp Biol Med 2005: accepted for publication.

[97] Frielingsdorf J, Deseo T, Gerber AE, Bertel O. A comparison of quality-of-life in patients with dual chamber pacemakers and individually programmed atrioventricular delays. Pacing Clin Electrophysiol 1996; 19(8): 1147–1154.

[98] Furlan R, Piazza S, Dell'Orto S, et al. Cardiac Autonomic Patterns Preceding Occasional Vasovagal Reactions in Healthy Humans. Circ 1998;98: 1756–1761.

[99] Garcia-Civera R, Ruiz-Granell R, Morell-Cabedo S, Sanjuan-Manez R, Perez-Alcala F, Plancha E, Navarro A, Botella S, Lacer A. Selective use of diagnostic tests in patients with syncope of unknown cause. JACC 2003;41:787–790.

[100] Gatzoulis KA, Mamarelis IE, Apostolopoulos T, Dilaveris P, Gialafos J, Toutouzas. Polymorphic ventricular tachycardia induced during tilt table testing in a patient with syncope and probable dysfunction of the sinus node. PACE 1995;18:1075–1079.

[101] Glickstein JS, Axelrod FB, Friedman D. Electrocardiographic repolarization abnormalities in familial dysautonomia: An indicator of cardiac autonomic dysfunction. Clin Auton Res 1999;9(2):109–112.

[102] Gradman A, Deedwania P, Cody R, Massie B, Packer M, Pitt B, Goldstein S, for the Captopril-Digoxin Study Group. Predictors of total mortality and sudden death in mild to moderate heart failure. J Am Coll Cardiol 1989;14:564–570.

[103] Gras D, Mabo P, Tang T, Luttikuis O, Chatoor R, Pedersen AK, Tscheliessnigg HH, Deharo JC, Puglisi A, Silvestre J, Kimber S, Ross H, Ravazzi A, Paul V, Skehan D. Multisite pacing as a supplemental treatment of congestive heart failure: preliminary results of the Medtronic Inc. InSync Study. Pacing Clin Electrophysiol 1998;21:2249–2255.

[104] Graux P, Mekerke W, Lemaire N, et al. Le syndrome du sinus carotidien. Apport de la monitorisation de la pression arterielle à l'exploration electrophysiologique endocavitaire. Arch Mal Coeur 1989;82:193–199.

[105] Greenfield ADM. An emotional faint. Lancet 1951;1:1302–1303.

[106] Griffin B, Shah P, Ferguson J, Rubin S. Incremental prognostic value of exercise hemodynamic variables in chronic congestive heart failure secondary to coronary artery disease or to dilated cardiomyopathy. Am J Cardiol 1991;67:848–853.

[107] Grubb B, Kosinski D. Tilt table testing: concepts and limitations. PACE 1997; 20:781–787.

[108] Grubb BP, Gerard G, Rousch K, et al. Differentiation of convulsive syncope and epilepsy with head up tilt table testing. Ann Intern Med 1991;115:871–876.

[109] Grubb BP, Gerard G, Roush K, et al. Cerebral vasoconstriction during head upright tilt-induced vasovagal syncope. A paradoxical and unexplained response. Circulation 1991;84:1157–64.

[110] Grubb BP, Gerard G, Wolfe DA, Samoil D, Davenport CW, Homan RW. Syncope and seizure of psychogenic origin: Identification with head-upright tilt table testing. Clin Cardiol 1992;15:839–842.

[111] Grubb BP, Hunt C, Samoil D, et al. Provocation of bradycardia and hypotension by head upright tilt table testing in survivors of the sudden infant death syndrome. PACE 1993;16:892.

[112] Grubb BP, Karas B. Diagnosis and management of neurocardiogenic syncope. Curr Opinion Cardiol 1998;13:29–35.

[113] Grubb BP, Klingenheben T: Posturales orthostatisches Tachykardiesyndrom (POTS): Ätiologie, Diagnose und Therapie. Med Klin 2000;95:442–446.

[114] Grubb BP, Kosinski D, Pothoulakis AJ. New and emerging indications for head upright tilt table testing. Eur J Cardiac Pacing Electrophysiol 1995;5:109–112.

[115] Grubb BP, Kosinski D. Serotonin and syncope: an emerging connection? Eur J Cardiac Pacing Electrophysiol 1996;5:306–14.

[116] Grubb BP, Kosinski DJ, Boehm K, et al. The postural orthostatic tachycardia syndrome. A neurocardiogenic variant identified during head-up tilt table testing. PACE 1997;20:2205–2212.

[117] Grubb BP, Rubin AM, Wolfe D, Temesy-Armos P, Hahn H, Elliott L. Head upright tilt table testing: a useful tool in the evaluation of recurrent vertigo of unknown origin associated with neurocardiogenic syncope or syncope. Otolaryngol Head Neck Surg 1992;107:570 –575.

[118] Grubb BP, Temesy-Armos P, Hahn H, Elliott L. Utility of upright tilt table testing in the evaluation and management of syncope of unknown origin. Am J Med 1991;90:6–10.

[119] Grubb BP, Temesy-Armos P, Moore J, et al. The use of head-up tilt table testing in the evaluation and management of syncope in children and adolescents. PACE 1992;15:742–748.

[120] Grubb BP, Wolfe D, Samoil D, et al. Recurrent unexplained syncope in the elderly: the use of head-upright tilt table testing in evaluation and management. J Am Geriatr Soc 1992;40:1123–1128.

[121] Grubb BP, Wolfe D, Samoil D, Temesy-Annos P, Hahn H, Elliott L. Usefulness of fluoxetine hydrochloride for prevention of resistant upright tilt induced syncope. PACE 1993;16:458–464.

[122] Grubb BP, Wolfe W, Temesy-Armos, P, Hahn H, Elliott L. Reproducibility of head upright tilt table test results in patients with syncope. PACE 1992;15:1477–1481.

[123] Grubb PB, Samoil D. Neurocardiogenic syncope. In: Kenny RA, ed. Syncope in the older patient: causes, investigations and consequences of syncope and falls. London: Chapmann and Hall 1996:1–106.

[124] Gullberg B, Johnell O, Kanis JA. World-wide projections for hip fracture. Osteoporosis Int 1997;7:407–413.
[125] Guzzetti S, Cogliati C, Turiel M, et al. Sympathetic predominance followed by functional denervation in the progression of chronic heart failure. Eur Heart J 1995;16:1100–1107.
[126] Hachul D, Scanavacca M, Sosa E. Does a role exist for tilting-guided therapy in the management of neurocardiogenic syncope? Arq Bras Cardiol 2002;78(2):167–171.
[127] Hachul D, Sosa E, Cansolim F, et al. Valor diagnóstico do teste de inclinação na avaliação da síncope de origem indeterminada: resultados preliminares. Arq Bras Cardiol 1994;62:7–9.
[128] Hadase M, Azuma A, Zen K, Asada S, Kawasaki T, Kamitani T, Kawasaki S, Sugihara H, Matsubara H. Very low frequency power of heart rate variability is a powerful predictor of clinical prognosis in patients with congestive heart failure. Circ J. 2004;68(4):343–347.
[129] Hainsworth R. Syncope: what is the trigger? Heart 2003;89:123–124.
[130] Hammill SC, Holmes DR, Wood DL. Electrophysiologic testing in the upright position: improved evaluation of patients with rhythm disturbance using a tilt table. J Am Coll Cardiol 1984;4:65–71.
[131] Hoefnagels WAJ, Padberg GW, Overweg J, et al. Transient loss of consciousness: the value of the history for distinguishing seizure from syncope. J Neurol 1991;238:39–43.
[132] Hon EH, Lee ST. Electronic evaluations of the fetal heart rate patterns preceding fetal death: further observations. Am J Obstet Gynecol 1965;87:814–826.
[133] Huang SKS, Ezri MD, Honser RG, Denes P. Carotid sinus hypersensitivity in patients with unexplained syncope: clinical, electrophysiologic, and long-term follow-up observation. Am Heart J 1988;116:989–996.
[134] Hull SS Jr, Vanoli E, Adamson PB, Verrier RL, Foreman RD, Schwartz PJ. Exercise training confers anticipatory protection from sudden death during acute myocardial ischemia. Circulation 1994;89:548–552.
[135] Iskos D, Dutton J, Scheinman MM, Lurie KG. Usefulness of pindolol in neurocardiogenic syncope. Am J Cardiol 1998;82:1121–1124.
[136] Ismer B, Von Knorre GH, Voss W, Grille W, Klenke G, Pulya K, Koglek W, Suntinger A, Luessow H. Exercise induced sympathetic influences do not change interatrial conduction times in VDD and DDD pacing. Pacing Clin Electrophysiol 1996;19:1786–1790.
[137] Jacob G, Costa F, Shannon J-R, et al. The neuropathic postural tachycardia syndrome. N Engl J Med 2000;343:1008–1014.

[138] Jaeger FJ, Schneider L, Maloney JD, Cruse RP, Fouad-Tarazi FM. Vasovagal syncope: role of head-up tilt test in patients with positive ocular compression test. PACE 1990;13:1416–1423.
[139] Jhamb DK, Singh B, Sharda B, et al. Comparative study of the efficacy of metoprolol and verapamil in patients with syncope and positive head-up tilt test response. Am Heart J 1996;132:608–6011.
[140] Kapoor W, Fortunato M, Hanusa BH, Schulberg HC. Psychiatrie illnesses in patients with syncope. Am J Med 1995;99:505–512.
[141] Kapoor W, Karpf M, Wieand S, Peterson J, Levey G. A prospective evaluation and follow-up of patients with syncope. N Engl J Med 1983;309:197–204.
[142] Kapoor W. Evaluation and outcome of patients with syncope. Medicine (Baltimore) 1990;69:160–175.
[143] Kapoor WN. Syncope. New Engl J Med 2000;343:1856–1862.
[144] Kapoor WN, Brant N. Evaluation of syncope by upright tilt testing with isoproterenol. A nonspecific test. Ann Intern Med 1992;116:358–363.
[145] Kapoor WN, Hanusa B. Is syncope a risk factor for poor outcomes? Comparison of patients with and without syncope. Am J Med 1996;100: 646–655.
[146] Kapoor WN, Peterson J, Wieand HS, Karpf M. Diagnostic and prognostic implications of recurrences in patients with syncope. Am J Med 1987;83: 700–708.
[147] Kapoor WN, Smith M, Miller NL. Upright tilt testing in evaluating syncope: a comprehensive literature review. Am J Med 1994;97:78–88.
[148] Kardos A, Watterich G, de Menezes R, Csanády M, Casadei B, Rudas L. Determinants of spontaneous baroreflex sensitivity in a healthy working population. Hypertension 2001;37:911–916.
[149] Kaufmann H. Neurally mediated syncope and syncope due to autonomic failure: differences and similiarities. J Clin Neurophysiol 1997;14:183–196.
[150] Kelly T, Cremo R, Nielson C, Shabetai R. Prediction of outcome in late-stage cardiomyopathy. Am Heart J 1990;119:1111–1121.
[151] Kenny RA, Bayliss J, Ingram A, Sutton R. Head up tilt: a useful test for investigating unexplained syncope. Lancet 1986;1:1352–1354.
[152] Kenny RA, McIntosh SJ. Carotid sinus syndrome. In: Kenny RA, ed. Syncope in the older patient: causes, investigations and consequences of syncope and falls. London: Chapman & Hall 1996:107–122.
[153] Kenny RA, O'Shea D, Parry SW. The Newcastle protocols for head-up tilt table testing in the diagnosis of vasovagal syncope, carotid sinus hypersensitivity and related disorders, Heart 2000;83:5 564–569.

[154] Kenny RA, O'Shea D, Walker HF. Impact of a dedicated syncope and falls facility for older adults on emergency beds. Age and Ageing 2002;31: 272–275.

[155] Keogh A, Baron D, Hickie J. Prognostic guides in patients with idiopathic or ischemic dilated cardiomyopathy assessed for cardiac transplantation. Am J Cardiol 1990;65:903–908.

[156] Khurana RK, Nicholas EM Head-up tilt test: How far and how long? Clin Auton Res 1996;6:335–341.

[157] Kleiger RE, Miller JP, Bigger JT Jr, Moss AJ, and the Multicenter Post-Infarction Research Group. Decreased heart rate variability and its association with increased mortality after acute myocardial infarction. Am J Cardiol 1987;89:256–262.

[158] Koizumi K, Kollai M. Control of reciprocal and non-reciprocal action of vagal and sympathetic efferents: study of centrally induced reactions. J Auton Nerv Syst 1981;3:483–501.

[159] Kolb HJ, Böhm U, Rother T, et al. Assessment of the optimal atrioventricular delay in patients with dual chamber pacemakers using impedance cardiography and doppler echocardiography. J Clin Basic Cardiol 1999;2:237.

[160] König U, Linzer M, Pontinen M, Divine GW. Syncope in young adults: evidence for a combined medical and Psychiatric approach. J Intern Med 1992;232:169–176.

[161] Krahn AD, Klein GJ, Norris C, Yee R. The etiology of syncope in patients with negative tilt table and electrophysiological testing. Circulation 1995;92:1819–1824.

[162] Krahn AD, Klein GJ, Yee R, et al. Randomized assessment of syncope trial: conventional diagnostic testing versus a prolonged monitoring strategy. Circulation 2001;104:46–51.

[163] Krahn AD, Klein GJ, Yee R, Takle-Newhouse T, Norris C. Use of an extended monitoring strategy in patients with problematic syncope. Circulation 1999;99:406–410.

[164] Krediet P, van Dijk N, Linzer M, et al. Management of vasovagal syncope: controlling or aborting faints by leg crossing and muscle tensing. Circulation 2002;106:1684–1689.

[165] Kubicek WG, Karnegis JN, Patterson BP, Witsoe DA, Mattson RH. Development and evaluation of an impedance cardiac output system. Aerospace Med 1936;87:1208–1212.

[166] KubiceK WG, Patterson RP, Witsoe DA. Impedance cardiography is a non-invasive method of monitoring cardiac function and other parameters of the cardiovascular system. Ann NY Acad Sci 1970;170,724–732.

[167] Kubicek WG, Witsoe DA, Patterson HP, From AHL. Development and evaluation of an impedance cardiographic system to measure cardiac output and other cardiac parameters. Final Progress Report to the National Aeronautics and Space Administration 1970.

[168] La Rovere MT, Bigger JT Jr, Marcus FI, Mortara A, Schwartz PJ. Baroreflex sensitivity and heart-rate variability in prediction of total cardiac mortality after myocardial infarction. ATRAMI (Autonomic Tone and Reflexes After Myocardial Infarction) Investigators. Lancet 1998;351(9101): 478–484.

[169] La Rovere MT, Mortara A, Pantaneleo P, Maestri R, Cobelli F, Tavazzi L. Scopolamine improves autonomic balance in advanced congestive heart failure. Circulation 1994;90:838–843.

[170] La Rovere MT, Mortara A, Pinna GD, et al. Quantification of baroreflex sensitivity by FINAPRES in patients after myocardial infarction: the ATRAMI experience. J Am Coll Cardiol 1997;29:470.

[171] La Rovere MT, Mortara A, Schwartz PJ. Baroreflex sensitivity. J Cardiovasc Electrophysiol 1995;6:761–774.

[172] La Rovere MT, Pinna GD, Maestri R, Mortara A, Capomolla S, Febo O, Ferrari R, Franchini M, Gnemmi M, Opasich C, Riccardi PG, Traversi E, Cobelli F Short-term heart rate variability strongly predicts sudden cardiac death in chronic heart failure patients, Circulation 2003;107: 565–570.

[173] La Rovere MT, Specchia G, Mortara A, Schwartz PJ. Baroretlex sensitivity, clinical correlates and cardiovascular mortality among patients with an early myocardial infarction: a prospective study. Circulation 1988;78: 816–824.

[174] Lasater M, Von Rueden KT. Outpatient cardiovascular management utilizing impedance cardiography. AACN Clin Issues 2003;14(2):240–250.

[175] Leman RB, Clarke E, Gillette P. Significant complications can occur with ischemic heart disease and tilt table testing.PACE 1999;22:675–677.

[176] Lempert T, Bauer M, Schmidt D. Syncope: a videometric analysis of 56 episodes of transient cerebral hypoxia. Ann Neurol 1994;36:233–237.

[177] Lenk M, Alehan, Ozme S, Celiker A, Ozer S. The role of serotonin re-uptake inhibitors in preventing recurrent unex≠plained childhood syncope – a preliminary report. Eur J Pediat 1997;156:747–750.

[178] Lerman-Sagie T, Rechavia E, Strasberg B, Sagie A, Blieden L, Mimouni M. Head-up tilt for the evaluation of syncope of unknown origin in children. J Pediatr 1991;118:676–679.

[179] Levy MN, Schwark PJ, eds. Vagal control of the heart: experimental basis and clinical implications. Armonk NY: Futura Publishing Co, 1994.

[180] Lewis T. A lecture on vasovagal syncope and the carotid sinus mechanism with comments on Gower's and Nothnagel's syndrome. Br Med J 1932;1: 873–876

[181] Likoff MJ, Chandler S, Kay H. Clinical determinants of mortality in chronic congestive heart failure secondary to idiopathic dilated or to ischemic cardiomyopathy. Am J Cardiol 1987;59:634–638.

[182] Linde C, Leclercq C, Rex S, Garrigue S, Lavergne T, Cazeau S, McKenna W, Fitzgerald M, Deharo JC, Alonso C, Walker S, Braunschweig F, Bailleul C, Daubert JC. Long-term benefits of biventricular pacing in congestive heart failure: results from the MUltisite STimulation in cardiomyopathy (MUSTIC) study.J Am Coll Cardiol. 2002;40(1):111–118.

[183] Linzer M, Felder A, Hackel A, Perry AJ, Varia I, Melville ML. Psychiatric syncope: a new look at an old disease. Psychosomatics 1990;31:181–188.

[184] Linzer M, Pritchett ELC, Pontinen M, McCarthy E, Divine GW. Incremental diagnostic yield of loop electrocardiographic recorders in unexplained syncope. Am J Cardiol 1990;66:214–219.

[185] Linzer M, Yang EH, Estes NA III, Wang P, Vorperian VR, Kapoor WN. Diagnosing syncope. 1. Value of history, physical examination, and eletrocardiography: Clinical Efficacy Assessment Project of the American College of Physicians. Ann Intern Med 1997;127:76–86.

[186] Lord SW, Clayton RH, Hall MCS, Gray JC, Murray A, McComb JM, Kenny RA. Reproducibility of three different methods of measuring baroreflex sensitivity in normal subjects. Clinical Science 1998;95:575–581.

[187] Low P, Bannister R. Multiple system atrophy and pure autonomic failure. In: Low P. Clinical Autonomic Disorders. Philadelphia, PA: Lippincott-Raven, 1997:555–575.

[188] Low PA, Opfer-Gehrking TL, Textor SC et al. Postural tachycardia syndrome (POTS). Neurology 1995;45(suppl 5):19–25.

[189] Lown B, Verrier RL. Neural activity and ventricular fibrillation. N Engl J Med 1976;294:1165–1170.

[190] Ludbrook J. Haemorrhage and shock. In: Hainsworth R, Mark A L, eds. Cardiovascular reflex control in health and disease. London: Saunders, 1993:463–490.

[191] Lurie KG, Benditt D. Syncope and the autonomic nervous system. J Cardiovasc Electrophysiol 1996;7:760–776.

[192] Mabo P, Ritter P, Varin C, Kermarrec A, Leclercq C, Bedossa M, Daubert C. Value of an algorithm of automatic adaptation of the atrio-ventricular delay to the instantaneous atrial rate in cardiac stimulation. Arch Mal Coeur Vaiss 1992;85(7):1001–1009.

[193] Madigan NP. Flaker GC. Curtis JJ, Reid J. Mueller KJ. Murphy TJ. Carotid sinus hypersensitivtiy: Beneficial effects of dual-chamber pacing. Am J Cardiol 1984;53:1034–1010.

[194] Madrid A, Qrtega I. Rebollo GJ, et al. Lack of efficacy of atenolol for the prevention of neurally-mediated syncope in highly symptomatic population: a prospective double-blind, randomized and placebo-controlled study. J Am Coll Cardiol 2001;37:554–557.

[195] Madsen B, Keller N, Christiansen E, Christensen N. Prognostic value of plasma catecholamines, plasma renin activity, and plasma atrial natriuretic peptide at rest and during exercise in congestive heart failure: comparison with clinical evaluation, ejection fraction, and exercise capacity. J Cardiac Failure 1995;1:207–216.

[196] Maggioni AP, Zuanetti G, Franzosi MG, et al. Prevalence and prognostic significance of ventricular arrhythmias after acute myocardial infarction in the fibrinolytic era: GISSI-2 results. Circulation 1993;87:12–22.

[197] Mahanonda N, Bhuripanyo K, Kangkagate C, et al. Randomized double-blind, placebo-controlled trial of oral atenolol in patients with unexplained syncope and positive upright tilt table test results. Am Heart J 1995;130:1250–1253.

[198] Malik M, Camm AJ. Significance of long-term components of heart rate variability for the further prognosis after acute myocardial infarction. Cardiovasc Res 1990;24:793–803.

[199] Malik M, Farrell T, Camm AJ. Circadian rhythm of heart rate variability after acute myocardial infarction and its influence on the prognostic value of heart rate variability. Am J Cardiol 1990;66:1049–1054.

[200] Malik M, Farrell T, Cripps T, Camm AJ. Heart rate variability in relation to prognosis after myocardial infarction: selection of optimal processing techniques. Eur Heart J 1989;10:1060–1074.

[201] Malliani A, Lombardi F, Pagani M, Cerutti S. Power spectral analysis of cardiovascular variability in patients at risk for sudden cardiac death. J Cardiovasc Electrophysiol 1994;5(3):274–286.

[202] Malliani A, Lombardi F, Pagani M. Power spectral analysis of heart rate variability: a tool to explore neural regulatory mechanisms. Br Heart J 1994;71:1–2.

[203] Malliani A, Recordati G, Schwartz PJ. Nervous activity of afferent cardiac sympathetic fibres with atrial and ventricular endings. J Physiol (Lond) 1973;229:457–469.

[204] Markush RE, Karp HR, Heyman A, O'Fallon WM. Epidemiologic study of migraine symptoms in young women. Neurol 1975;25:430–5.

[205] Maron B, Shirani J, Poliac L, et al. Sudden death in young competitive athletes: clinical, demographic and pathologic profiles. JAMA 1996;276: 199–204.
[206] Marti B, Villiger B, Hintermann M, Lerch R. Plötzlicher Herztod beim Sport: Sinnvolle Vorsorgeuntersuchungen und Präventionsmassnahmen, Schweizerische Zeitschrift für Sportmedizin und Sporttraumatologie 1998;46:83–85.
[207] Martin GJ, Adams SL, Martin HG, Mathews J, Zull D, Scanlon PJ. Prospective evaluation of syncope. Ann Emerg Med 1984;13:499–504.
[208] Martin TP, Hanusa BH, Kapoor WN. Risk stratification of patients with syncope. Ann Emerg Med 1997;29:459–466.
[209] Mathias C. Autonomic disorders and their recognition. New Engl J Med 1997;336:721–724.
[210] McHarg ML, Shinnar S, Rascoff H, Walsh CA. Syncope in childhood. Pediatr Cardiol 1997;18:367–371.
[211] McIntosh SJ, Lawson J, Kenny RA. Clinical characteristics of vasodepressor, cardioinhibitory and mixed carotid sinus syndrome in the elderly. Am J Med 1993;95:203–208.
[212] McKenna, Deanfield J, Faraqui A, England D, Oakley C, Goodwin J. Prognosis in hypertrophic cardiomyopathy: role of age and clinical, electrocardiographic and hemodynamic features. Am J Cardiol 1981;47: 532–538.
[213] Menozzi C, Brignole M, Lolli G, et al. Follow-up of asystolic episodes in patients with cardioinhibitory, neurally mediated syncope and VVI pacemaker. Am J Cardiol 1993; 72:1152–1155.
[214] Middlekauff H, Stevenson W, Stevenson L, Saxon L. Syncope in advanced heart failure: high risk of sudden death regardless of origin of syncope. J Am Coll Cardiol 1993;21:110–116.
[215] Milstein S, Buetikofer J, Dunnigan A, Benditt DG, Gornick C, Reyes WJ. Usefulness of disopyramide for prevention of upright tilt-induced hypotension-bradycardia. Am J Cardiol 1990;65:1339–1344.
[216] Moak JP, Bailey JJ, Makhlouf FT. Simultaneous heart rate and blood pressure variability analysis: insight into mechanisms underlying neurally mediated cardiac syncope in children. J Am Coll Cardiol 2002;40;8: 1466–1474.
[217] Morichetti A, Astorino G. Epidemiological and clinical findings in 697 syncope events. Minerva Medica 1998;89:211–220.
[218] Morillo CA, Eckberg DL, Ellenbogen KA, Beightol LA, Hoag JB, Tahvanainen KUO, Kuusela TA, Diedrich AM. Vagal and sympathetic mechanisms in patients with orthostatic vasovagal syncope. Circulation 1997;96:2509–2513.

[219] Morillo CA, Klein GJ, Gersh BJ. Can serial tilt testing be used to evaluate therapy in neurally mediated syncope? Am J Cardiol 1996;77:521–523.

[220] Morillo CA, Klein GJ, Jones DL, Yee R. Time and frequency domain analyses of heart rate variability during orthostatic stress in patients with unexplained neurally mediated syncope. Am J Cardiol 1994;74: 1258–1262.

[221] Morillo CA, Klein GJ, Zandri S, Yee R. Diagnostic accuracy of a low-dose isoproterenol head-up tilt protocol. Am Heart J 1995;129:901–906.

[222] Morillo CA, Leitch JW, Yee R, Klein GJ. A placebo-controlled trial of intravenous and oral disopyramide for prevention of neurally mediated syncope induced by head up tilt. Am J Cardiol 1993;22:1843–1848.

[223] Morley CA, Perrins EJ, Grant PL, Chan SL, McBrien DJ, Sutton R. Carotid sinus syncope treated by pacing. Analysis of persistent symptoms and role of atrioventricular sequential pacing. Br Heart J 1982;47:411–418.

[224] Morley CA, Sutton R. Carotid sinus syncope. Int J Cardiol 1984;4: 287–293.

[225] Mortara A, La Rovere MT, Signorini MG, et al. Can power spectral analysis of heart rate variability identify a high risk subgroup of congestive heart failure patients with excessive sympathetic activation? A pilot study before and after heart transplantation. Br Heart J 1994;71: 422–430.

[226] Mosqueda-Garcia R, Furlan R, Fernandez-Violante R. Sympathetic and baroreceptor reflex function in neurally mediated syncope evoked by tilt. J Clin Invest 1997;99(11):2736–2744.

[227] Moya A, Brignole M, Menozzi C, et al. Mechanism of syncope in patients with isolated syncope and in patients with tilt-positive syncope. Circulation 2001;104:1261–1267.

[228] Moya A, Permanyer-Miralda G, Sagrista-Sauleda J, et al. Limitations of head-up tilt test for evaluating the efficacy of therapeutic interventions in patients with vasovagal syncope: results of a controlled study of etilefrine versus placebo. J Am Coll Cardiol 1995;25:65–69.

[229] Mtinangi BL, Hainsworth R. Increased orthostatic tolerance following moderate exercise training in patients with unexplained syncope. Heart 1998;80:596–600.

[230] Muller G, Deal B, Strasburger JF, Benson DW Jr. Usefulness of metoprolol for unexplained syncope and positive response to tilt testing in young persons. Am J Cardiol 1993;71:592–595.

[231] Munro NC, McIntosh S, Lawson L, et al. Incidence of complications after carotid sinus massage in older patients with syncope. J Am Geriatr Soc 1994;42:1248–1251.

[232] Naschitz JE, Gaitini L,Mazov L, et al. The capnography-tilt test for the diagnosis of hyperventilation syncope.Q J Med 1997;90:139–145.
[233] Natale A, Akhtar M, Jazayeri M, et al. Provocation of hypotension during head-up tilt testing in subjects with no history of syncope or presyncope. Circulation 1995;92:54–58.
[234] Natale A, Geiger MJ, Maglio C, Newby KN, Dhala A, Akhtar M, Sra J. Recurrence of neurocardiogenic syncope without pharmacologic interventions. Am J Cardiol 1996;77:1001–1003.
[235] Natale A, Sra J, Akhtar M, et al. Use of sublingual nitroglycerin in patients with unexplained syncope. Am Heart J 1998;135:564–570.
[236] Niederlag W, Lüderitz B, Hempel A, Lemke H. Telekardiologie. Health Academy 01/2004.
[237] Nino J, Villar JC, Tahvanainen KUO, Kahonen M, Kuusela TA, Morillo CA. Vasovagal susceptibility to nitrate or isoproterenol head-up tilt. Am J Cardiol 2001;88:1326–1330.
[238] Notarius CF, Butler GC, Ando S, et al. Dissociation between microneurographic and heart rate variability estimates of sympathetic tone in normal subjects and patients with heart failure. Clin Sci 1999;96: 557–565.
[239] Novak L, Penaz J, Kotovskaya AR, Vil-Vilyams IF, Lukjanuk VJu, Nikolashin GF. Perspectives for the application of the Penaz's method for a non-invasive continuous blood pressure measurement in space medicine. Physiologist. 1991;34:230–231.
[240] Nyboer J, Bagno S, Barnett A, Halsey RH. Radiocardiograms – the electrical impedance changes of the heart in relation to electrocardiograms and heart sounds. Amer Soc Clin 1940;19:773.
[241] Nyboer J. Electrical impedance plethysmography. Springfleld 1969. III: 243 pp.
[242] Nyman JA, Krahn AD, Bland PC, Griffiths S, Manda V. The costs of recurrent syncope of unknown origin in elderly patients. Pacing Clin Electrophysiol 1999;22:1386–1394.
[243] O'Mahoney D. Pathophysiology of carotid sinus hypersensitivity in elderly patients. Lancet 1995;346:950–952
[244] O'Connor GT, Collins R, Burning JE, et al. Rehabilitation with exercise after myocardial infarction. Circulation 1989;82:234–244.
[245] Oberg B, Thoren P. Increased activity in left ventricular receptors during haemorrhage or occlusion of caval veins in the cat. A possible cause of the vasovagal reaction. Acta Physiol Scand 1972;85:164–173.
[246] Occhetta E, Bortnik M, Audoglio R, Vassanelli C. Closed loop stimulation in prevention of vasovagal syncope. Inotropy controlled pacing in

vasovagal syncope (INVASY): a multicentre randomized, single blind, controlled study. Europace 2004;6:538–547.
[247] Occhetta E, Bortnik M, Vassanelli C. The DDDR closed loop stimulation fort he prevention of vasovagal syncope: results from the INVASY prospective feasibility registry. Europace 2003;5:153–162.
[248] Odemuyiwa O, Malik M, Farrell T, Bashir Y, Poloniecki J, Camm J. Comparison of the predictive characteristics of heart rate variability index and left ventricular ejection fraction for all-cause mortality, arrhythmic events and sudden death after acute myocardial infarction. Am J Cardiol 1991;68:434–439.
[249] Oraii S, Maleki M, Minooii M, Kafai I. Comparing two different protocols for tilt table testing: sublingual glyceryl trinitrate versus isoprenaline infusions. Heart 1999;81:603–605.
[250] Parameshwar J, Keegan J, Sparrow J, Sutton G, Poole-Wilson P. Predictors of prognosis in severe chronic heart failure. Am Heart J 1992;123: 421–426.
[251] Parati D, Di Renzo M, Bertinieri G. Evaluation of the baroreceptor-heart reflex by 24-hour intra-arterial blood pressure monitoring in humans. Hypertension. 1988;12:214–222.
[252] Parati G, Di Rienzo M, Macia G. How to measure baroreflex sensitivity: from the cardiovascular laboratory to daily life. J Hypertens 2000;18: 7–19.
[253] Parati G, Omboni S, Frattola A, Di Rienzo M., Zanchetti A, Mancia G. Evaluation of the baroreflex in ambulant subjects. IOS Press 1992: 123–137.
[254] Parati G, Ongaro G, Bilo G, Glavina F, Castiglioni P, Di Rienzo M, Mancia G. Non-invasive beat-to-beat blood pressure monitoring: new developments. Blood Press Monit 2003;8(1):31–36.
[255] Parry SW, Kenny RA The managment of vasovagal syncope, QJ Med 1999;92:697–705.
[256] Parry SW, Richardson DA, O'Shea D, et al. Diagnosis of carotid sinus hypersensitivity in older adults: carotid sinus massage in the upright position is essential. Heart 2000;83:22–23.
[257] Penaz J, Honzikova N, Fiser B. Spectral analysis of resting variability of some circulatory parameters in man. Physiol Bohemoslov 1978;27(4): 349–357.
[258] Penaz J. Criteria for set point estimation in the volume clamp method of blood pressure measurement. Physiol Res. 1992;41(1):5–10.
[259] Petersen MEV, Chamberlain-Webber R, Fizpatrick AP, Ingram A, Williams T, Sutton R. Permanent pacing for cardioinhibitory malignant vasovagal syndromc. Br Heart J 1994;71:274–281.

[260] Petersen MEV, Price D, Williams T, Jensen N, Riff K, Sutton R. Short AV interval VDD pacing does not prevent tilt induced vasovagal syncope in patients with cardioinhibitory vasovagal syndrome. PACE 1994;17: 882–891

[261] Pitzalis M, Parati G, Massari F, Guida P, Di Rienzo M, Rizzon B, Castiglioni P, Iacoviello M, Mastropasqua F, Rizzon P. Enhanced reflex response to baroreceptor deactivation in subjects with tilt-induced syncope. J Am Coll Card 2003;41(7):1167–1173.

[262] Pongiglione G, Fish F, Strasburger JF, Benson DW. Heart rate and blood pressure response to upright tilt in patients with unexplained syncope. J Am Coll Cardiol 1990;16:165–170.

[263] Raschke C, Parzeller M, Kind M, Banzer W. Organpathologische Ursachen des akuten Sporttodes in Deutschland, Österreich und der deutschsprachigen Schweiz. Dt Z Sportmed 1998;49:157–160.

[264] Raviele A, Brignole M, Sutton R, et al. Effect of etilefrine in preventing syncopal recurrence in patients with vasovagal syncope: a double-blind, randomized, placebo-controlled trial. The Vasovagal Syncope International Study. Circulation 1999;99:1452–1457.

[265] Raviele A, Gasparini G, Di Pede F, et al. Nitroglycerin infusion during upright tilt: a new test for the diagnosis of vasovagal syncope. Am Heart J 1994;127:103–111.

[266] Raviele A, Gasparini G, DiPede F, Delise P, Bonso A, Piccolo E. Usefulness of head-up tilt test in evaluating patients with syncope of unknown origin and negative electrophysiologic study. Am J Cardiol 1990;65: 1322–1327.

[267] Raviele A, Giada F, Brignole M, et al. Diagnostic accuracy of sublingual nitroglycerin test and low-dose isoproterenol test in patients with unexplained syncope. A comparative study. Am J Cardiol 2000;85: 1194–1198.

[268] Raviele A, Giada F, Menozzi C, Speca G, Orazi S, Gasparini G, Sutton R, Brignole M; Vasovagal Syncope and Pacing Trial Investigators. A randomized, double-blind, placebo-controlled study of permanent cardiac pacing for the treatment of recurrent tilt-induced vasovagal syncope. The vasovagal syncope and pacing trial (SYNPACE). Eur Heart J 2004;25(19):1741–1748.

[269] Raviele A, Proclemer A, Gasparhini G, et al. Long-term follow-up of patients with unexplained syncope and negative etectrophysiologic study. Eur Heart J 1989;10:127–132.

[270] Raviele SA, Menozzi C, Brignole M, et al. Value of head-up tilt testing potentiated with sublingual nitroglycerin to assess the origin of unexplained syncope. Am J Cardiol 1995;76:267–272.

[271] Reybrouck T, Heidbuchel H, Van De Werf F, et al. Long-term folluw-up results of tilt-training therapy in patients with recurrent neurocardiogenic syncope. Pacing Clin Electrophysiol 2002;25:1441–1446.

[272] Robertson DA, Taylor R. Metabolic and endocrine causes of syncope. In: Kenny RA, ed. Syncope in the older patient: causes, investigations and consequences of syncope and falls. London: Chapman & Hall 1996: 240–265.

[273] Rockman H, Juneau C, Chatterjee K, Rouleau J-L. Long-term predictors of sudden and low output death in chronic congestive heart failure secondary to coronary artery disease. Am J Cardiol 1989;64:1344–1348.

[274] Ross BA, Hughes S, Anderson E, Gillette PC. Abnormal responses to orthostatic testing in children and adolescents with recurrent unexplained syncope. Am Heart J 1991;122:748 –754.

[275] Ross J, Braunwald E. Aortic stenosis. Circulation 1968;38:61–67.

[276] Rossen R, Kabat H, Anderson JP. Acute arrest of cerebral circulation in man. Arch Neurol Psychiatr 1943;50:510–528.

[277] Rowe PC, Bou-Holaigah I, Kan J, Calkins H. Is neurally-mediated hypotension an unrecognized cause of chronic fatigue? Lancet 1995;345: 623–624.

[278] Rushmer, BF, Christal DK, Wagner C, Ellis RM. Intracardiac impedance plethysmography. Amer J Phys 1953;174:171.

[279] Samniah N, Sakaguchi S, Ermis C, Lurie KG, Benditt DG. Transient modification of baroreceptor response during tilt-induced vasovagal syncope. Europace 2004;6:48–54.

[280] Samoil D, Grub BP, Brewster P, Moore J, Temesy-Armos P. Comparison of single and dual chamber pacing techniques in prevention of upright tilt induced vasovagal syncope. Eur J Cardiac Pacing Electrophysio! 1993;1: 36–41.

[281] Sandrone G, Mortara A, Torzillo D, La Rovere MT, Malliani A, Lombardi F. Effects of beta blockers (atenolol or metoprolol) on heart rate variability after acute myocardial infarction. Am J Cardiol 1994;74:340–345.

[282] Savage DD, Corwin L, McGee DL, Kanell WB, Wolf PA. Epidemiologic features of isolated syncope: the Framingham Study. Stroke 1985;16: 626–629.

[283] Scherrer U, Vissing S, Morgan BJ, Hanson P, Victor RG. Vasovagal syncope after infusion of a vasodilatator in a heart transplant recipient. N Engl J Med 1990;322:602–604.

[284] Schwartz PJ, Billman GE, Stone HL. Autonomic mechanisms in ventricular fibrillation induced by myocardial ischemia during exercise in dogs with

healed myocardial infarction: an experimental preparation for sudden cardiac death. Circulation 1984;69:790–800.

[285] Schwartz PJ, Pagani M, Lombardi F, Malliani A, Brown AM. A cardiocardiac sympathovagal reflex in the cat. Circ Res 1973;32:215–222.

[286] Schwartz PJ, Priori SG. Sympathetic nervous system and cardiac arrhythmias. In: Zipes DP, Jalife J, eds. Cardiac electrophysiology: from cell to bedside. Philadelphia: WB Saunders Co, 1990:330–343.

[287] Schwartz PJ, Vanoli E, Stramba-Badiale M, De Ferrari GM, Billman GE, Foreman RD. Autonomic mechanisms and sudden death: new insights from analysis of baroreceptor reflexes in conscious dogs with and without a myocardial infarction. Circulation 1988;78:969–979.

[288] Seller H. Central baroreceptor reflex pathways. In: Persson PB, Kirchheim IIR, eds. Baroreceptor Reflexes. Berlin: Springer Verlag, 1991:45–74

[289] Shaley Y, Gal R, Tchou PJ, Anderson AJ, Avitall B, Akhtar M, et al. Echocardiographic demonstration of decreased left ventricular dimensions and vigorous myocardial contraction during syncope induced by head-up tilt. J Am Coll Cardiol 1991;18:46–51.

[290] Sheldon R, Killam S. Methodology of isoproterenol-tilt table testing in patients with syncope. J Am Coll Cardiol 1992;19:773–779.

[291] Silvani S, Padoan G, Guidi AR, Bianchedi G, Maresta A. Cerebral vasoconstriction in neurally mediated syncope: relationship with type of head-up tilt test response. Ital Heart J. 2003;4:768–775.

[292] Silverstein MD, Singer DE, Mulley AG, Thibault GE, Barnett GO. Patients with syncope admitted to medical intensive care units. JAMA 1982;248: 1185–1189.

[293] Sleight P, La Rovere MT, Mortara A, et al. Physiology and pathophysiology of heart rate and blood pressure variability in humans: is power spectral analysis largely an index of baroreflex gain? Clin Sci 1995;88:103–109.

[294] Smit AAJ, Halliwill JR, Low PA, Wieling W. Topical Review. Pathophysiological basis of orthostatic hypotension in autonomic failure. J Physiol 1999;519:1–10.

[295] Smith ML, Ellenbogen KA, Eckberg DL. Sympathoinhibition and hypotension in carotis sinus hypersensitivity. Clin Aut Res 1992;2:389–392

[296] Soteriades ES, Evans JC, Larson MG, et al. Incidence and prognosis of syncope. N Engl J Med 2002;347:878–875.

[297] Sra J, Andersen A, Sheikh S, et al. Unexplained syncope evaluated by ectrophysiologic studies and head-up tilt testing. Ann Intern Med 1991;114:1013–1019.

[298] Sra J, Maglio C, Biehl M, Dhala A, et al. Efficacy of midodrine hydrochloride in neurocardiogenic syncope refractory to standard therapy. J Cardiovasc Electrophysiol 1997;8:42–46.

[299] Sra JS, Jazayeri MR, Avitall B, Dhale A, Desphande S, Blanck Z, Akhtar M. Comparison of cardiac pacing with drug therapy in the treatment of neurocardiogenic (vasovagal) syncope with bradycardia or asystole. N Engl J Med 1993;328:1085–1090.

[300] Sramek BB. Measurement of cardiac output in pregnancy by thermodilution and impedence techniques. Br J Obstet Gynaecol 1990;97(1): 90–92.

[301] Stevens PM. Cardiovascular dynamics during orthostatsis and the influence of intravascular instrumentation. AM J Cardiol 1966;17:211–218.

[302] Stevenson L, Couper G, Natterson B, Fonarow G, Hamilton M, Woo M, Creaser J. Target heart failure populations for new therapies. Circulation 1995;92(suppl II):II-174–II-181.

[303] Strasberg B, Rechavia E, Sagie A, et al. The head-up tilt table test in patients with syncope of unknown origin. Am Heart J 1989;118:923–927.

[304] Sugrue DD, Gersh BJ, Holmes DR, Wood DL, Osborn MJ, Hammill SC. Symptomatic ‚isolated' carotid sinus hyper-sensitivity: Natural history and results of treatment with anticholinergic drugs or pacemaker. J Am Coll Cardiol 1986;7:158–162.

[305] Sutton R, Brignole M, Menozzi C, Raviele A, Alboni P, Giani P, Moya A. Dual-chamber pacing in the treatment of neurally mediated tilt-positive cardioinhibitory syncope: pacemaker versus no therapy: a multicenter randomized study. The Vasovagal Syncope International Study (VASIS) Investigators. Circulation 2000;102(3):294–299.

[306] Sutton R, Petersen M, Brignole M, Raviele A, Menozzi C, Giani P. Proposed classification for tilt induced vasovagal syncope. Eur J Cardiac Pacing Electrophysiol 1992;3:180–18.

[307] Task Force of the European Society of Cardiology and the North American Society of Pacing and Electrophysiology. Heart rate variability: standards of measurement, physiological interpretation and clinical use. Circulation 1996;93:1043–1065; Eur Heart J 1996;17:354–381.

[308] The CONTAK CD Investigators. Cardiac resynchronisation therapy in heart failure (CONTAK-CD) clinical study. Presented at the meeting of the North American Society of Pacing Electrophysiologists, Boston, 2001.

[309] The Multicenter Postinfarction Research Group. Risk stratification and survival after myocardial infarction. N Engl J Med 1983;309:331–336.

[310] Thilenius OG, Quinones JA, Husayni TS, Novak J. Tilt test for diagnosis of unexplained syncope in pediatric patients. Pediatrics 1991;87:334–338.

[311] Thomas JE. Hyperactive carotis sinus reflex and carotid sinus syncope. Mayo Clin Proc 1969;44:127–139.

[312] Tonkin AL, Frewin DB. Drugs, toxins and chemicals that alter autonomic function. In: Mathias CJ, Bannister R, eds. Autonomic failure. 4th edn. Oxford: Oxford University Press 1999:527–533.
[313] Tonnesen G, Haft J, Fulton J, Rubenstein D. The value of tilt testing with isoproterenol in determining therapy in adults with syncope and presyncope of unexplained origin. Arch Intern Med 1994;154:1613–1617.
[314] UK Department of Health: National Service Framework for Older People, Standard Six: Falls 2001. http://www.doh.gov.uk/nsf/olderpeople.htm.
[315] Unverferth D, Magorien R, Moeschberger M, Baker P, Fetters J, Leier C. Factors influencing the one-year mortality of dilated cardiomyopathy. Am J Cardiol 1984;54:147–152.
[316] Van de Borne P, Montano N, Pagani M, et al. Absence of low-frequency variability of sympathetic nerve activity in severe heart failure. Circulation 1997;95:1449–1454.
[317] Van der Meer BJ, Woltjer HH, Sousman AM, Schreuder WO, Bulder ER, Huybregts MA, de Vries PM. Impedance cardiography. Importance of the equation and the electrode configuration.Intensive Care Med 1996 Oct;22(10):1120–1124.
[318] Vanoli E, De Ferrari GM, Stramba-Badiale M, Hull SS Jr, Foreman RD, Schwartz PJ. Vagal stimulation and prevention of sudden death in conscious dogs with a healed myocardial infarction Circ Res 1991;68(5): 1471–1481.
[319] Vink A, Erbas T. Recognizing and treating diabetic autonomic neuropathy. Cleve Clin J Med 2001;68:928–944.
[320] Volkmann H, Schnerch B, Kuhnert H. Diagnostic value of carotid sinus hypersensitivity. PACE 1990;13:2065–2070.
[321] Volpi A, De Vita C, Franzosi MG, et al. Determinants of 6-month mortality in survivors of myocardial infarction after thrombolysis: results of the GISSI-2 data base. Circulation 1993;88:416–4129.
[322] Ward CR, Gray JC, Gilroy JJ, Kenny RA. Midodrine: a role in the management of neurocardiogenic syncope. Heart 1998;79:45–49.
[323] Waxman MB, Yao L, Cameron DA, Wald RW, Roseman J. Isoproterenol induction of vasodepressor-type reaction in vasodepressor-prone persons. Am J Cardiol 1989;63;58–65.
[324] Weiling W, Smith AAJ, De Jong-De Vos Van Steenwijk CCE, Van Lieshout JJ, Karemaker JM. Pathophysiological mechanisms underlying vasovagal syncope in young subjects. Pacing Clin Electrophysiol 1997;20:2034–2038.
[325] Wesseling KH. Finger arterial pressure measurement with Finapres. Z Kardiol 1996;85(Suppl3):38–44.

[326] Whitehorn, WV, Perl ER. The use of change in capacity to record cardiac volume in human subjects. Science 1949;108:262–283.

[327] Wolf MM, Varigos GA, Hunt D, Sloman JG. Sinus arrhythmia in acute myocardial infarction. Med J Aust 1978;2:52–53.

[328] Wright C, Drinkhill M J, Hainsworth R. Reflex effects of independent stimulation of coronary and left ventricular mechanoreceptors in anaesthetized dogs. J Physiol 2000;528:349–358.

[329] Wu TC, Hachul D, Scanavacca M, Sosa M. Diagnostic value of the tilt-table test for the assessment of syncope in children and adolescents. Arq Bras Cardiol 2001;77:505–508.

[330] Young JB, Abraham WT, Smith AL, Leon AR, Lieberman R, Wilkoff B, Canby RC, Schroeder JS, Liem LB, Hall S, Wheelan K; Multicenter InSync ICD Randomized Clinical Evaluation (MIRACLE ICD) Trial Investigators. Combined cardiac resynchronization and implantable cardioversion defibrillation in advanced chronic heart failure: the MIRACLE ICD Trial. JAMA. 2003;289(20):2685–2694.

[331] Youosazi AK, Franklin WH, Chan DP, Cassidy SC, Allen HD. Oral fluid therapy. A promising treatment for vasodepressor syncope. Arch Pediatr Adolesc Med 1998;152:165–168.

[332] Zabel M, Klingenheben T, Hohnloser SH. Changes in autonomic tone following thrombolytic therapy for acute myocardial infarction: assessment by analysis of heart rate variability. J Cardiovasc Electrophysiol 1994;5:211–218.

[333] Zaidi A, Clough P, Scheepers B, Fitzpatrick A. Treatment resistant epilepsy or convulsive syncope. BMJ 1998;317:869–870.

[334] Ziegler D. Cardiovascular autonomic neuropathy: clinical manifestations and measurement. Diabetes Rev 1999;7:342–357.

[335] Ziemssen T, Süss M, Reichmann H. Die kardiovaskuläre Funktionsdiagnostik des autonomen Nervensystems – eine Einführung. Neurophysiol Lab 2002;24/2:57–77.

Subject index